50
Simple Ways
to Pamper
Yourself

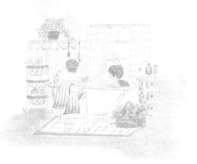

The mission of Storey Communications is to serve our customers by publishing practical information that encourages personal independence in harmony with the environment.

Edited by Deborah Balmuth and Robin Catalano
Cover design by Meredith Maker
Cover and interior illustrations by Carleen Powell
Text design and production by Mary B. Minella
Indexed by Susan Olason, Indexes & Knowledge Maps

The information in this book is true and complete to the best of our knowledge. All recommendations are made without guarantee on the part of the author or Storey Books. The author and publisher disclaim any liability in connection with the use of this information. For additional information, please contact Storey Books, Schoolhouse Road, Pownal, Vermont 05261.

Storey books are available for special premium and promotional uses and for customized editions. For further information, please call Storey's Custom Publishing Department at 1-800-793-9396.

Printed in the United States by R.R. Donnelley
10 9 8 7 6 5 4 3 2 1

Library of Congress Cataloging-in-Publication Data

Tourles, Stephanie L., 1962–
    50 simple ways to pamper yourself / Stephanie Tourles.
      p. cm.
    ISBN 1-58017-210-5 (pbk. : alk. paper)
    1. Beauty, Personal.   2. Herbal cosmetics.   3. Health.   I.
Title.   II. Title: Fifty simple ways to pamper yourself
  RA778.T637   1999
    613—dc21   99-33055
                                            CIP

50
Simple Ways
to Pamper
Yourself

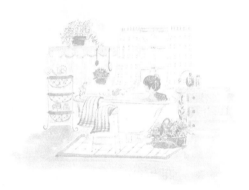

Stephanie Tourles

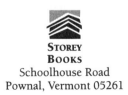

STOREY BOOKS
Schoolhouse Road
Pownal, Vermont 05261

Contents

Dedication

To my husband, Bill . . . thanks for your strong
shoulders, your never-ending support,
your laughter, your encouragement to explore
my dreams, to push my limits, to find my life's
direction. I love you more and more with
each breath I take, my sweet William.

Acknowledgments

All books start with an idea, a seed. I wish to thank
my editor, Deborah Balmuth, for giving me this seed
and asking me to fertilize it and make it grow. And
many thanks to those of you who most graciously
shared with me your favorite ways to pamper your-
selves and improve your health and well-being.

Let Go of the Guilt

T he word *pamper* is a verb meaning "to gratify the wishes of, especially by catering to physical comforts." It also means "to spoil, coddle, humor, indulge, or caress." Sounds like pampering is something most of us could use more of in these stressful times.

If you bought this book for yourself, did you feel just a little bit guilty buying a book devoted solely to pampering? Are you afraid that someone will think you're being selfish by wanting to spend some quality time dedicated to boosting your own well-being? Well, chase those thoughts right out of your head. Don't think of pampering yourself as decadence or forbidden pleasure. Think of it as a way to preserve your sanity in an insanely paced world.

We're all so very busy, busy, busy. Buzzing around like worker bees, tending to everyone else's needs and ignoring our own, to a large extent. Do you work all day caring for children or elderly parents, or work outside the home in a 40- to 60-hour-per-week career? Are you a full-time student? Isn't it pure ecstasy to know that after you finish all that work, you get to go grocery shopping, cook dinner, do the laundry, clean the house, pay the bills, mow the lawn, fix the car, and meet with the insurance agent? Sure it is! Who needs personal time?

As if life wasn't busy enough before technology exploded onto the scene, now we're expected to be super-people. Living life at breakneck speed can make us feel as if we're on a wild roller-coaster ride that won't stop. We can't continue to work faster and faster and process more and more information and still function as normal, happy, healthy human beings. Needless to say, most of us are frazzled. We need a break … to catch our breath, to regain our health, to restore our natural rhythms, to enjoy the meaningful moments in life that have gone by the wayside because we're so busy. In a word, we need *pampering*.

It's not a dirty word that should make you feel guilty. You deserve a bit of pampering. I'm sure you've earned it.

By pampering yourself, you don't have to take an entire day off and loaf around (though that's advisable from time to time); you can simply integrate small moments of pampering into your everyday life. This book is filled with simple ways to de-stress and unwind, to find more pleasure, more joy, and to look and feel better about your-self. These invaluable tips will help you enjoy more "you" time. When you're happier and calmer, radiant from the inside out, glowing with health and beauty, believe me, those around you will sit up and take notice.

INFORMATION AND CAUTIONS

Most of the ingredients mentioned in this book, including essential oils and herbs, can be found in natural-food or health-food stores. Natural product and herbal mail-order suppliers are also a good place to look.

When using any new ingredient for the first time, it's always best to try a patch test. Apply a bit of the ingredient or formula to the inside of your arm, and allow it to remain for 24 hours. If any signs of allergic response — redness, itching, or other skin irritation — occur, discontinue use immediately. In addition, be sure to use caution in handling pure essential oils. Because they are highly concentrated, they can cause adverse skin reactions. Always use a dropper when measuring essential oils, and do not use more than recommended; more can be dangerous, not better. Keep all ingredients out of the reach of children and pets.

So go ahead, pamper yourself . . . you're worth it!

Blessings of health and happiness to you and yours,

Stephanie L. Tourles

C'mon Get Happy

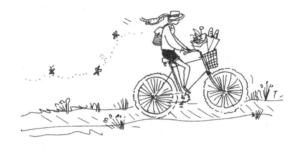

R emember how you danced and sang as a child, usually in a group of other smiling, laughing children? Can you remember how everyone looked: clear-eyed, with radiant faces and glowing health? Recapture this youthful happiness and low level of stress and you are guaranteed to feel better.

As an added bonus, you'll even look better. Why? Stress restricts blood flow to the skin, preventing moisture and nutrients from getting where they need to go. Stress also promotes the production of the male hormone testosterone, which stimulates oil production. That, in turn, promotes pimple formation and clogged pores. Lowering your stress level will dramatically improve the texture and condition of your skin.

Manage Your Stress

Use lavender essential oil to help you relax; it is a natural sedative and nervine. When I'm about to give a speech and herbal demonstration to a group of people, I still, to this day, get quite nervous. To regain my confident and calm demeanor, I place 3 drops of pure lavender essential oil onto a soft tissue or small handkerchief and inhale deeply of the floral aroma about five times just prior to my presentation. I'm serene within minutes.

Job or family demands getting to you? This exercise sequence works wonders to help you refocus, de-stress, and re-energize:

- Stand up with your feet shoulder width apart, placing your palms on your lower abdomen. Close your eyes and slowly inhale through your nose, gradually expanding your diaphragm. If you're breathing correctly, you will feel your hands move outward. Hold for a count of five, then exhale slowly through your mouth. Do this 10 times.

- Now that you're calmer and have more oxygen circulating throughout your body, place your arms straight out in front of you. Slowly do 10 deep knee bends. Make sure to squeeze your buttocks on the way back up. Don't you feel better now?

Smile more. Even if you're having a bad day, try to find at least one good thing that will bring a smile to your face. Is the sky bright and sunny? Are the birds singing? Are you healthy? Is there fresh snow on the ground? Do you have a beautiful manicure?

Laugh more. "Laughter is the best medicine" — how true that is. Go see a funny movie, read a funny book, play with your children (children are always laughing), or play with your pet. Laughter makes you feel good, makes your skin glow, and stimulates circulation throughout your body. Go ahead — have a good, hearty guffaw!

Get-Happy Herb Tea

When you're at your wit's end and your nerves are jangling, make a cup or two of this soothing, relaxing tea. Happiness and peace of mind are only minutes away. All the herbs in this recipe are dried.

     2 cups boiling water
     ½ teaspoon lemon balm leaves
     ½ teaspoon chamomile flowers
     ½ teaspoon lavender flowers
     ¼ teaspoon passionflower leaves or flowers
     ½ teaspoon spearmint or peppermint leaves

Remove the pot of boiling water from the heat, add the herbs, cover, and steep for 5 to 10 minutes. Strain. Add honey or lemon to taste, if desired. Sip slowly and enjoy! This tea is also delicious iced for a refreshing summer beverage.

Get Steamed

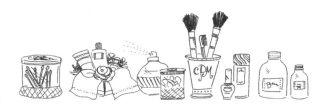

An herbal facial steam will hydrate your skin and allow your pores to perspire and breathe. As the steam penetrates your skin, the various herbs will soften its surface, act as an astringent, and aid in healing skin lesions. Also, any clogging from dirt or makeup will be loosened for easy removal afterward.

Herbal steams can be used regularly by those with normal, dry, or oily skin. Those of you with sensitive skin, dilated capillaries, rosacea, or sunburned skin, however, should abstain. Always cleanse your skin before steaming.

Steams for Pore Perfection

To prepare a facial steam, boil 4 cups of distilled water (and vinegar, if the recipe calls for it). Remove from the heat, add herbs, cover, and allow to steep for about 5 minutes. Place the pot in a safe, stable place where you can sit comfortably for about 10 minutes. Use a bath towel to create a tent over your head, shoulders, and steaming herb pot; allow 10 to 12 inches between the steaming herb pot and your face to avoid burning your skin. Close your eyes, breathe deeply, and relax.

All the herbs in the following blends are in dried form. If you're using fresh herbs, double the quantity.

For Normal or Oily Skin: 1 teaspoon yarrow, 1 teaspoon sage, 1 teaspoon rosemary, and 1 teaspoon peppermint.

For Normal or Dry Skin: 1 teaspoon orange flowers, 2 teaspoons comfrey leaves, and 1 teaspoon elder flowers.

For All Skin Types: 1 teaspoon calendula, 1 teaspoon chamomile, 1 teaspoon raspberry leaves, 1 teaspoon peppermint, and 1 teaspoon strawberry leaves.

Wrinkle Chaser: 1 tablespoon crushed fennel seeds and 2 drops essential oil of rose or rose geranium. Add the essential oil to the water immediately before you steam your face.

Aromatherapy to Relax or Recharge

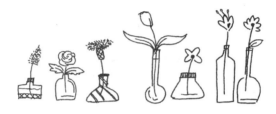

The word *aroma,* meaning "a pleasant or agreeable odor arising from spices, plants, or flowers," combined with the word *therapy,* or "the remedial treatment of a disease or other physical or mental disorder," gives us the true definition of the word *aromatherapy:* a healing modality that involves the use of aromatic essences or essential oils of plants.

Incorporating essential oils into your life is a pleasurable way to enhance your physical, emotional, and spiritual well-being. Aromatherapy can beautify your complexion, reduce stress, stimulate creativity, lull you to sleep, and pep you up, as well as help heal severe burns and reduce scar formation.

Strike a Balance

One of the easiest and most pleasant ways to benefit from aromatherapy is in the bath. At day's end, add 3 to 6 drops of your favorite gentle essential oil, such as lavender, Roman or German chamomile, or clary sage, to a full tub of water and swish with your hands to blend. Slip into the water and breathe deeply. Relax …

Intensify the potency of your peppermint tea. Give it a little zing by adding 1 or 2 drops of essential oil of peppermint. Inhale the invigorating steam. This tea is super for a midmorning pick-me-up, or to relieve a stuffy head or case of indigestion. Makes your breath minty-fresh, too!

To ease the pain of muscle cramps, sore tendons, arthritis, or overexertion in general, the clean, fresh, lemony scent of essential oil of *Eucalyptus citriodora* makes a soothing addition to massage oil. Add 10 to 15 drops of essential oil to ½ cup of almond, hazelnut, grapeseed, or soybean oil, mix well, and massage away the discomfort. Enlist the help of a partner or good friend if possible, and promise to return the favor.

Harmony Aroma Oil

This formula can be adjusted to suit your particular emotional and physical needs. You may want to create all three versions so that you'll have the appropriate one on hand when you need it. Caution: These formulas are for inhalation only. Do not apply directly to the skin; they may cause irritation.

> 1 tablespoon pure, unrefined almond, jojoba, or hazelnut oil
>
> 1 of the following blends:
>
> **Calming Blend:** For excess stress, restlessness, or trouble sleeping, or if the weather outside is cold and dry, add ½ teaspoon lavender, ½ teaspoon neroli, ½ teaspoon clary sage, and ½ teaspoon bergamot essential oils.
>
> **Cooling Blend:** For times of irritability, impatience, fiery disposition, or chaos, or if the weather outside is hot and uncomfortable and your skin is extra sensitive and itchy, add ½ teaspoon lavender, ½ teaspoon jasmine, ½ teaspoon Roman chamomile, and ½ teaspoon spearmint essential oils.
>
> **Stimulating Blend:** If you're feeling slow and lethargic, in need of an energetic lift, and maybe a bit congested, or if the weather is dreary, cool, and damp, add ½ teaspoon cinnamon, ½ teaspoon orange, ½ teaspoon ginger, and ½ teaspoon cypress essential oils.

Combine the base oil with the blend of your choice in a 2-ounce, dark-colored glass bottle and cap tightly. The blend needs one week to synergize and develop, so shake your formula vigorously twice daily for seven days. After one week, place a few drops on a soft handkerchief or tissue and inhale the comforting herbal aroma as needed. The aroma can also be inhaled directly from the bottle.

Make a Splash

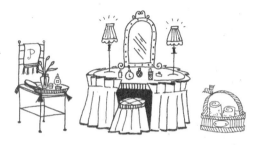

Nothing is more cooling and invigorating to hot summer skin than a chilled splash or spritz of a freshly made, fragrant natural skin toner. Like a summer breeze that soothes your parched skin and revives your senses, these lightly scented toners can be customized to your particular skin type and fragrance preference.

Give Your Skin a "Drink"

Natural skin toners have been used for centuries to refresh, pamper, and gently scent the skin and air. The following toner recipes can be applied as a splash, a light mist from a spray bottle, or with cotton balls. Use at any time of the day or immediately after cleansing to remove traces of cleanser and prepare your skin for moisturizer. Store in the refrigerator and discard after one week unless otherwise indicated.

For normal or oily skin, brew a cup of strong peppermint or lemon balm tea. Chill it, and use it to remove excess oil and shine from your skin.

For itchy, rashy skin, pour a cup of boiling water over 1 teaspoon of crushed fennel seeds. Steep for 10 minutes. Strain and chill.

For all skin types, brew a cup of strong chamomile tea, chill, and use to soften and moisturize. This is particularly good to use during the winter, when skin dehydrates and chaps easily.

For normal and dry skin, add 1 tablespoon of vegetable glycerin to ½ cup of rose water. The glycerin will act as a humectant and draw water vapor from the air to your skin. This makes a super, light floral summer moisturizer that can be stored in the refrigerator for up to six months. Shake before each use.

Polish Your Body

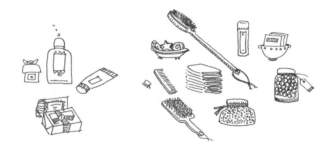

A cosmetic scrub is used to remove dry, dead cells from the surface of the skin. It can be used on all skin types except those with acne, thread (spider) veins, or extreme sensitivity; a scrub may be too irritating for such conditions. These recipes will leave your skin softer, sleeker, and more refined, in prime condition to absorb an application of moisturizer.

Natural Scrubs and Salt Rubs

For dry and/or sensitive skin: In a small bowl, combine 1 tablespoon of instant, powdered whole milk, 1 scant tablespoon of ground oatmeal, and enough water to form a spreadable paste. Allow to thicken for 1 minute. Massage onto your face and throat, avoiding the eye area. Rinse. This formula may be used daily in place of soap to gently cleanse your face and body. It will not irritate or dry your skin.

Especially for men or those with thick, oily skin: In a small bowl, combine 1 teaspoon of ground oatmeal, 1 teaspoon of finely ground almond meal, 1 teaspoon of fine sea salt, and ½ teaspoon of powdered peppermint or rosemary leaves with enough of your favorite herbal astringent to form a spreadable paste. Allow to thicken for 1 minute. Massage gently onto your face and throat, avoiding the eye area. Rinse. This blend is particularly good to use on the chest, back, or shoulders if minor pimple breakouts tend to occur.

For all skin types: In a small bowl, combine ¼ cup sea salt (or plain sugar) with ¼ cup of warmed coconut or olive oil. Stir together. Gently massage onto your body with your hands or a mitt using light but firm pressure. Continue massaging until a rosy glow appears. Rinse with warm water, then towel-dry. This blend is beneficial for those suffering from severely dry skin: It will effectively remove the top layer of dead skin cells, allowing for proper moisturizer absorption. *Note:* This scrub should not be used on your face or immediately after shaving any area of your body; it could cause stinging and irritation.

For all skin types, especially dehydrated: In a small bowl, combine 1 tablespoon of finely ground sunflower seed meal with 1 tablespoon of applesauce. Gently massage this paste onto your face and throat. Let it remain for 10 minutes so that the oils of the sunflower seeds can be released and absorbed into your thirsty skin. Rinse with warm water, and then pat dry.

GRINDING INGREDIENTS

In order to grind oatmeal, sunflower seeds, almonds, dried herbs, and similar ingredients, I like to use a regular coffee grinder specifically reserved for cosmetic making. A blender or food processor works well for batches larger than 1 cup. Either method will create a fine, powderlike consistency.

6

Step Lively

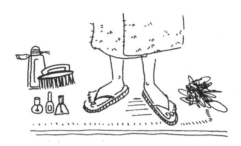

My feet are killing me!" Do you ever say that at the end of a long day? Whether you're a construction worker, athlete, secretary, stay-at-home parent, or fashion model, your feet take a lot of abuse. Most people stuff their feet into ill-fitting shoes and suffer from cramped and strained arches, heel pain, hammertoes, bunions, calluses, corns, and toe cramps.

If you want your feet to provide you with years of uninterrupted service, treat them with the utmost care. Daily hygiene and a few foot exercises go a long way toward this goal. Do keep in mind though, that 10 to 15 minutes of foot exercise every day will not do any good if you continue to wear ill-fitting shoes that constrict movement and force your feet into unnatural shapes.

Exercise Those "Dogs"

The following foot, ankle, and toe exercises can be performed anytime you feel the need to stretch and release tension. If you can't slip off your shoes discreetly during the day, then perform the exercises when you get home from work or finish your daily errands. Slip your body into something more comfortable and slip your feet out of something uncomfortable (your shoes). Relax and unwind. A nice cup of soothing herbal tea, sipped while you do your exercises, tastes especially good, hot or cold!

Footsie Roller Massage: Wooden footsie rollers have been around for many years. They come in all shapes and sizes, from single to double or triple rollers. Some are handheld, and others sit on the floor. I particularly like the kind with raised ridges going from one end to the other; these are both stimulating and relaxing to my feet. If you don't have a footsie roller, a wooden rolling pin can be used in a pinch. Simply place the footsie roller or rolling pin on the floor and, while bearing down comfortably, roll the entire length of your foot over the tool, back and forth. Repeat, concentrating on your arches. Do this for 5 to 10 minutes per foot. This exercise relieves fatigue and cramping, especially in your arches.

The Golf Ball Roll: This exercise is recommended by Carol Frey, M.D., director of the Orthopaedic Foot and Ankle Center in

Manhattan Beach, California. "Roll a golf ball under the ball of your foot for 2 minutes. This is a great massage for the bottom of the foot and is recommended for people with plantar fasciitis (heel pain), arch strain, or foot cramps."

Point and Flex: This is a great exercise to stretch and strengthen just about everything from your knees down. Sit on the floor, legs stretched out in front of you and palms facing down at your sides. Now point your toes as hard as you can and hold for 5 seconds; then flex your foot up as hard as you can and hold for 5 seconds. Repeat a total of 10 times. If you experience cramping, cut back on your repetitions and gradually work up to 10.

Rubber-Band Big Toe Stretches: This exercise is helpful if you suffer from bunions or toe cramps resulting from wearing improperly fitting shoes. This exercise is also recommended by Dr. Carol Frey. Either sit on the floor with your legs stretched out in front of you and your palms on the floor beside or behind you, or sit in a chair with your feet flat on the floor. Place a nice, thick, moderately stiff rubber band around your big toes and pull your feet away from each other. Hold for 5 to 10 seconds, and then relax. Repeat 10 to 20 times. If this hurts, or if you have arthritis or bunions in advanced stages, do only as many as you can. Gradually increase as your toes gain strength.

7

Nourish Your Hair

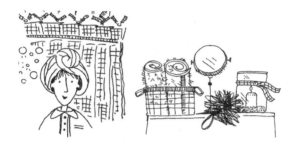

Healthy, shiny, bouncy hair is a reflection of proper nourishment and a healthy lifestyle. Even if you use the highest-quality natural shampoos, conditioners, and styling aids, the condition of your hair will still suffer if your diet is lacking in necessary nutrients. If your hair seems lackluster, try modifying your diet.

How to Have Healthy Hair

Eat more protein if your locks are limp, lifeless, and slow growing. Good sources of protein include eggs, lean meats and fish, beans and seeds, whole grains, and low-fat dairy or soy products.

Get your ABCs. These vitamins are vital to the health of your hair and scalp. Good sources of vitamin A include cod liver oil; red, yellow, and orange vegetables and fruits; spirulina; egg yolks; and deep green leafy vegetables. Good sources of vitamin C include citrus fruits, deep green leafy vegetables, rose hips, tomatoes, berries, pineapple, apples, persimmons, cherries, bell and hot peppers, papayas, and currants. Good sources of vitamin B include lean beef, poultry, egg yolks, liver, milk, brewer's yeast, whole grains, alfalfa, nuts and seeds, soy products, deep green leafy vegetables, spirulina, wheat germ, molasses, peas, and beans.

Cut back on caffeine, alcohol, refined sugar and flour, and junky snacks. These empty-calorie foods deplete your body's stores of vitamins B and C.

Include iodine, sulfur, zinc, and silica in your diet. These four minerals are essential for proper hair health. Good sources of iodine include all types of fish, spirulina, sunflower seeds, iodized salt, and sea salt. Good sources of sulfur include turnips, dandelion greens, radishes, horseradish, string beans, onions, garlic, cabbage, celery, kale, watercress, fish, lean meats, eggs, and asparagus. Good sources of zinc include spirulina, barley grass, alfalfa, kelp, wheat germ, pumpkin seeds, whole grains, brewer's yeast, milk, eggs, oysters, nuts, and beans. Good sources of silica include horsetail, spirulina, nettles, dandelion root, alfalfa, kelp, flaxseeds, oat straw, barley grass, wheat grass, apples, berries, burdock roots, beets, onions, almonds, sunflower seeds, and grapes.

Rapunzel's Favorite Herb Tea

Now, I won't guarantee that this tea will make you sprout hair as long and lush as Rapunzel's, but this mineral-rich brew is a delightful way to nourish your hair from the inside out. This recipe uses dried herbs, and will yield 2 cups of tea.

½ teaspoon horsetail
½ teaspoon raspberry leaves
½ teaspoon nettles
½ teaspoon oat straw
1 teaspoon peppermint
2 cups boiling water
Honey or lemon to taste (optional)

Add the herbs to the boiling water, then remove from heat. Cover and steep for 5 to 10 minutes. Strain. Add honey or lemon to taste, if desired. Sip slowly and enjoy!

8

Top 10 Healing Foods

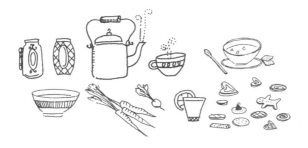

If you really want to pamper your mind and body, then partaking of these top 10 nutritionally dynamic foods is just what the doctor ordered. They'll help balance your moods; restore your energy; increase your stamina; nourish your hair, skin, and nails; and boost your immune system. They're delicious to boot!

Eat for Vibrant Health

Beans, beans, the magical food — the more you eat them, the better your mood! It's true: **Beans** are high in the B vitamins, known mood stabilizers. They're also high in complex carbohydrates, magnesium, iron, zinc, and fiber. A cup or so a day is recommended.

A cruciferous wonder, **broccoli** is a nutritional powerhouse. Just ½ cup several times per week delivers most of your daily required vitamin C, a dollop of vitamin A and the B complex, and plenty of minerals, especially calcium and magnesium; it's also rich in fiber.

The juicy, sweet **orange** is chock-full of skin-healthy, cold-fighting vitamin C, soluble and insoluble fiber, bioflavonoids, folate, and potassium. Consume one or more per day.

Apples are tasty, easy to carry, and thirst quenching. They're rich in soluble and insoluble fiber, potassium, and trace minerals. An apple a day sure won't hurt!

High in natural sugar, ripe **bananas** are self-contained packages of quick, healthy energy. They contain a fair amount of B-complex vitamins, vitamin C, and soluble and insoluble fibers, but are a good source of potassium and magnesium. Consume a few of these energy-boosting fruits each week.

Water can temporarily give you a feeling of fullness, hydrate your skin, keep your organs operating smoothly, and flush toxins out of your body. Drink 8 to 12, 8-ounce glasses each day, depending upon your level of activity.

Bone up on **sesame seeds.** These tiny, crunchy seeds are little storehouses of highly absorbable calcium and magnesium. They're also high in fiber and trace minerals. Look in health food stores for raw, unhulled seeds or jars of sesame tahini (sesame paste). Two tablespoons per day of seeds or paste will make a major contribution toward your daily mineral requirement.

Want a lean, low-calorie food that delivers a powerful nutritional punch? Then reach for **shellfish.** Shrimp, scallops, clams, crab, abalone, lobster, snails, crayfish, oysters, conch, and prawns are high in beauty nutrients such as protein, B-complex vitamins, iron, iodine, zinc, and copper. Two servings per week are recommended.

Keep bacteria at bay and Dracula away by eating a clove or two of fresh **garlic** every day. This potent antioxidant can cut cholesterol, ward off infection, soothe a sore throat, protect your heart, and kill athlete's foot fungus. An ounce of fresh garlic contains a good helping of vitamin C, thiamin (vitamin B_1), potassium, sulfur, and iron.

Salmon is the king of flavor and a rich source of beneficial omega-3 fats, which have been determined to help prevent heart problems and lessen the symptoms of arthritis and PMS. One or more servings of salmon per week are recommended.

9

Five (Almost) Free Daily Rituals for Beautiful Skin

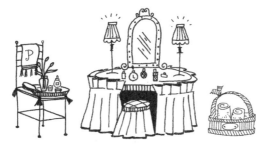

Skin care shouldn't be a complex chore. It should be simple, natural, and basic. And if a few of these straightforward skin-care rituals are free for the asking, then so much the better.

Tried-and-True Treatments

Cleansing Routine: A beauty must! Cleanse your skin twice daily (only once if your skin is dry) using a mild, natural, inexpensive cleanser designed for your skin type. Add a couple of drops essential oil of rose, spearmint, or orange to your cleanser to boost its cleaning effect and aromatic quality. Cleansing your skin is especially important before going to bed, because your body excretes toxins through your skin as you sleep. If facial pores are clogged with makeup and dirt, breakouts can occur. If you perspire a lot in your line of work or exercise heavily, then rinse off and massage your body with a coarse cloth or loofah before retiring to remove salt and dead-skin buildup. Your skin needs to breathe while you sleep!

Exercise: Try to exercise outside, to help oxygenate your cells with fresh air and facilitate waste removal through your skin. Exercises such as walking, biking, in-line skating, and weight lifting improve cardiovascular fitness and muscular endurance, which translates into increased energy and a rosy complexion. If you live in a city, try to find a green space — a park or a greenway — in which to exercise. If city streets, with their attendant pollution, are your only outdoor option, exercising in a gym may be a better alternative.

Sleep, Blissful Sleep: I don't care what else you do to your skin, if you are sleep deprived your skin will look sallow, dull, tired, and saggy; with your puffy eyes, you will resemble a frog prince or princess. And of course, your energy level will be less than desirable. Sleep: It's the best-kept skin-care secret there is!

Sunlight: Ten to 15 minutes unprotected exposure to sunlight several times a week is essential to the health of your bones and skin. It helps your body absorb calcium, due to the skin's ability to convert the sun's rays into vitamin D. Sun exposure helps heal eczema, psoriasis, and acne, and energizes your body. Plus those warm rays just make you feel good all over. If your dermatologist advises you to avoid the sun entirely, other sources of vitamin D include egg yolks, fish liver oil, vitamin-D-supplemented soy or cow's milk, organ meats, salmon, sardines, and herring.

Water: What goes in must go out, and water helps move everything along. Impurities not disposed of in a timely manner via the internal organs of elimination (such as the kidneys, liver, lungs, and large intestine) will find an alternate exit, namely your skin, sometimes referred to as the "third kidney." Pimples and rashes may develop as your body tries to unload its wastes through your skin. Eight to 12, 8-ounce glasses of pure water a day combined with a fibrous diet will help cleanse your body of toxins and keep your colon functioning as it should. Water also keeps your skin hydrated and moisturized, so drink up!

10

De-stress &
Relax

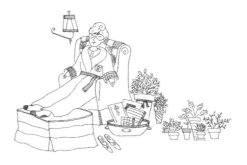

Seems like everyone is so very busy these days, no matter what their job description. I've spoken with many stay-at-home parents, career men and women, elderly folks, and students, asking them for their favorite methods to relax and de-stress after a hectic day. Try some of these ways to unwind.

Take a Load Off

"**If** I am stressed, I like to go for a long walk, because it helps me unwind."

"**If** stressed while at work, I try to breathe in deeply and then exhale slowly."

"I find taking a leisurely bath with oils or a bubble bath to be very soothing."

"To relax, I like doing stretching exercises for about 15 minutes or so with my eyes closed while listening to calming background music."

"My greatest de-stressor is usually a creative pursuit. I make quilts and garden, primarily. The final products are lasting delights that I cherish."

"I have a monthly facial."

"Cooking relaxes my mind and body. Eating what I've prepared is great, too!"

"Sipping a glass of wine while reading a good book chases the day's cares away."

"Good heart-to-heart conversation, a romantic candlelight dinner, and a walk on the beach at sunset with my husband is my idea of heaven."

"I like to putter in my garden, feel the soil, and pull weeds after work."

11

It's High Time for Tea

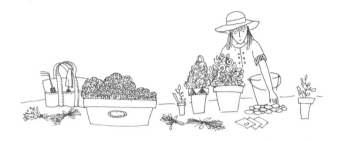

Nothing's more relaxing and refreshing than a good cup of herbal tea. Tea herbs are easily grown in pots or in your garden; all it takes are good soil, a sunny spot, water, compost or fertilizer, and a bit of TLC. Herb seeds for tea gardens are available in most garden centers or through seed catalogs. Follow seed-package directions for proper sowing, care, and harvesting.

For Your Sipping Pleasure

Plant one or all of the following easy-to-grow herbal tea blends. See the directions that follow for brewing the ultimate cup of tea from your fresh herbs. *Note:* Please be sure to use only organically raised herbs for culinary purposes; you don't want to ingest pesticides.

Lemon Lover's Blend: 2 teaspoons each lemon balm leaves, lemon verbena leaves, and lemon-grass leaves, plus fresh lemon juice to taste.

Mad about Mint: 2 teaspoons each peppermint leaves, spearmint leaves, and lemon mint leaves.

Licorice Delight: 2 teaspoons each fennel seeds, anise hyssop leaves, and cinnamon basil leaves.

Tension Ease: 2 teaspoons each chamomile flowers, lemon basil leaves, and raspberry leaves.

Fresh-n-Fruity: 2 teaspoons each pineapple mint leaves, orange mint leaves, apple mint leaves, and ginger mint leaves.

Cup-o-Calmness: 2 teaspoons each catnip leaves, lavender blossoms and leaves, rose petals, and lemon balm leaves.

Tea is wealth itself, because there is nothing that cannot be lost, no problem that will not disappear, no burden that will not float away, between the first sip and the last.

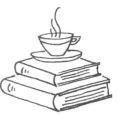

— Henry David Thoreau

The Ultimate Cup-o-Tea

For many people, brewing the perfect cup of tea is akin to art. Whether or not you agree, you're sure to enjoy a delicious, soothing cup of tea whenever the urge strikes. To make iced tea, double the amount of herbs called for in the recipe and brew as usual. Chill in the refrigerator and serve over ice when ready.

> Several cups purified, cool water
> 2 tablespoons herbal blend of choice (see opposite)

1. Bring the water to a rolling boil. Add 2 cups of the boiling water to a pottery, china, or glass teapot, swirl around, and leave for a few minutes to warm the pot.

2. For each cup of tea, place 2 tablespoons or so of fresh herbs into a tea ball or strainer. Empty the warm water out of the pot. Toss in the herb-filled tea ball or strainer and pour in the desired amount of boiling water. Cover and steep for 5 to 10 minutes.

3. Remove the herbs and strain if necessary; serve. Nice additions include lemon or orange juice, honey, sorghum syrup, maple syrup, stevia syrup, date sugar, soy milk, and cream.

Soothe Your Soles

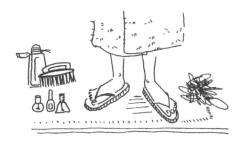

If your nerves are frayed, your energy level is running on empty, and your feet have seen better days, then by all means partake of an aromatherapy foot massage. It will soothe your spirits, reduce stress, put the spring back into your step, and soften your feet. What's good for the body is good for the "sole"!

Techniques of Foot Massage

Here are some standard foot-massage techniques that a professional nail technician might perform on a client during a pedicure. If you do not have a willing partner to give you a massage, never fear. These techniques are just as easily done by you on your own feet. Foot massage can be performed on dry or slightly oiled feet, using any vegetable oil and a drop or two of your favorite essential oil.

Step 1: Stroking stimulates circulation and warms the foot. Holding your partner's foot in your hands, on the top of the foot begin a long, slow, firm stroking motion with your thumbs, starting at the tips of the toes and sliding back away from you, all the way to the ankle; then retrace your steps back to the toes with a lighter stroke. Repeat this step three to five times. Now firmly stroke the bottom of the foot with your thumbs, starting at the base of the toes and moving from the ball of the foot over the arch, to the heel, and then back again. Repeat this step three to five times.

Step 2: Ankle rotations will loosen the joints and relax the feet. Cup one hand under the heel, behind the ankle, to brace the foot and leg. Grasp the ball of the foot with the other hand and turn the foot slowly at the ankle three to five times in each direction. With repeated foot massages, any stiffness will begin to recede. This is a particularly good exercise for those suffering from arthritis.

Step 3: Toe pulls and squeezes can be unbelievably calming, because toes are quite sensitive. Grasp the foot beneath the arch. With the other hand and beginning with the big toe, hold the toe with your thumb on top and index finger beneath. Starting at the base of the toe, slowly and firmly pull the toe, sliding your fingers to the top and back to the base. Now repeat, but gently squeeze and roll the toe between your thumb and index finger, working your way to the tip and back to the base. Repeat on the remaining toes.

Step 4: Toe slides are also very soothing. Grasp the foot behind the ankle, cupping under the heel. With the index finger of the other hand, insert your finger between the toes, sliding it back and forth three to five times.

Step 5: The arch press releases tension in the inner and outer longitudinal arches. Hold the foot as you did in step 4. Using the heel of your other hand, push hard as you slide along the arch from the ball of the foot toward the heel and back again. Repeat five times. This part of the foot can stand a little extra exertion, but don't apply too much pressure.

Step 6: Stroking is a good way to begin and end a foot massage. Repeat step 1, on page 35.

The way to health is to have an aromatic bath and a scented massage every day.

— **Hippocrates**

13

Take a Luxurious Milk Bath

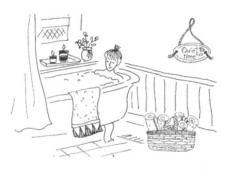

Why not use the skin-pampering benefits of milk by bathing in it instead of drinking it? Milk includes many components, such as proteins and fats, that are particularly good for soothing and moisturizing the skin.

Milk — for Softer, Sleeker Skin

To relieve itchy skin due to sunburn or poison ivy or oak irritation, add 1 cup of instant, powdered whole milk and 1 cup of baking soda to running bathwater. Step in and soak for 15 minutes.

Make a milk-bath bag. In a medium-size muslin drawstring bag or in a 12-inch square of doubled cheesecloth, place 1 cup of instant, powdered whole milk, ½ cup of borax, ¼ cup of ground lavender flowers, and ¼ cup of ground rose petals. Tie the ends together or wrap with an elastic band. Drop into the tub as it fills with water, step in, and rub the bag over your skin to soften and lightly scent.

To combat dry, super-sensitive skin or to bathe an infant's delicate skin, add 1 cup of instant, powdered whole milk, ¼ cup of finely ground raw almonds, pine nuts, walnuts, or pecans, and ¼ cup of marsh mallow root powder to a bath bag (see above). Drop into the tub as it fills with water, step in, and rub the bag over your skin.

Aromatherapeutic Milk Bath

Try this version of Cleopatra's famous bathing ritual and see if your skin doesn't feel softer and smoother.

- 1 cup instant, powdered whole goat's or cow's milk
- 1 tablespoon apricot kernel, jojoba, avocado, hazelnut, or extra-virgin olive oil
- 8 drops essential oil of German or Roman chamomile, lavender, rosemary, spearmint, or rose

Pour the powdered milk and oil together directly under running bathwater. Add the essential oil immediately before you step into the tub. Swish with your hands to mix. Now relax!

14

Cleanse & Condition Your Complexion

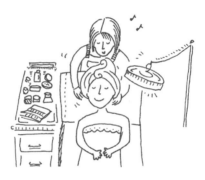

Simple, natural cleansing creams, fruit pastes, and grain blends can be used to effectively and economically remove makeup and everyday dirt and grime that collects in your pores. Unlike soap — which has a tendency to dry the skin's surface — these products are very gentle and nourishing and do a thorough job of cleansing without stripping your skin of its natural barrier of protective oils.

Restore the Radiance

For smooth, soft skin, wash your face every day with plain, organic yogurt or buttermilk. Use it as you would ordinary cold cream, avoiding the eye area. It's gentle enough for all skin types and as a bonus, it contains naturally occurring lactic acid. This acts as a mild exfoliant to remove dead-skin buildup.

For positively glowing skin, mash a third of a very, very ripe banana in a small bowl. Use the pulp to wash your face and throat, avoiding the eye area. If your skin is especially dry or dehydrated, leave this on for approximately 5 minutes. Rinse, then pat dry.

To pamper mature, thin, dry skin, mix 1 tablespoon of heavy cream with 1 or 2 drops of essential oil of rose or rose geranium. Use as you would a cleansing lotion, massaging well into your face and throat. This can be used on the eye area to remove eye makeup and mascara. This blend smells exquisite and if a drop happens to drip into your mouth, it will taste like a rose shake!

All-Purpose Cleanser

*This was my first-ever homemade cleansing formula —
created when I was 15! It's still my favorite recipe 21 years
later. It naturally cleanses skin of excess oils, makeup, and
dirt without drying, making it suitable for all skin types,
even sensitive. See the box on page 16 for information on
grinding ingredients.*

> ½ cup ground oatmeal
> ⅓ cup finely ground sunflower seeds
> ¼ cup finely ground almond meal
> 1 teaspoon powdered peppermint or rosemary
>   leaves, rose petals, or lavender flowers
> Dash cinnamon powder (optional)
> Water, 1 or 2 percent milk, or heavy cream to moisten

1. In a medium-size bowl, mix the dry ingredients together
thoroughly.

2. Using approximately 2 teaspoons of scrub mixture for
your face and throat, or more for your body, add enough
water (for oily skin), milk (for normal skin), or heavy cream
(for dry skin) to form a spreadable paste. Allow to thicken
for 1 minute. Massage onto your face and throat or body
area. Rinse.

3. Store any remaining blend in a zipper-lock plastic bag or
plastic food container in a cool, dry place for up to six
months, or up to a year in the freezer.

15

Keep Your Pearly Whites Gleaming

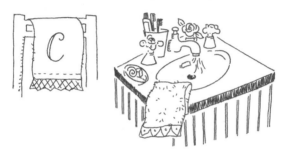

Most dentifrices available today contain harsh abrasives, saccharin, sugar, detergents, and bleaches. Combine these ingredients with the twice-daily use and misuse of toothbrushes and the result is tooth enamel and gum tissue suffering from extra wear and tear. You can make simple yet effective and pleasant-tasting natural dentifrices at home that will leave your teeth sparkling and your gums in the pink.

Step Back, Plaque

In a small bowl, combine 1 teaspoon of baking soda with 1 drop of essential oil of orange, lime, spearmint, or cinnamon. Dip a wet toothbrush into this mixture and brush your teeth as usual to fight plaque buildup and neutralize mouth odor.

Try strawberries for a brighter smile! Mash a very ripe strawberry into a pulp. Dip your toothbrush into the pulpy liquid and brush normally. Strawberries have a slight bleaching action. Rinse thoroughly after brushing.

Out on a weekend camping trip and forgot your toothbrush? Peel a 3- or 4-inch twig freshly cut from a sweet gum or flowering dogwood tree and chew on the end until it is frayed and soft. Now gently rub your teeth and gums. The twig can also be dipped in water and baking soda, if you desire.

Herbal Toothpaste

A great alternative to commercial sweetened toothpastes! This recipe yields about 10 applications.

- 4 teaspoons baking soda
- 1 teaspoon finely ground sea salt
- 1 teaspoon myrrh powder
- 1 teaspoon white cosmetic clay
- 2 tablespoons vegetable glycerin
- 10 drops essential oil of orange, tea tree, rosemary, anise, lemon, spearmint, or peppermint

In a small bowl, thoroughly blend all ingredients until a spreadable paste forms. Store in a small jar. Dip a dry toothbrush into the mixture and brush normally.

16

Find Time for Fitness

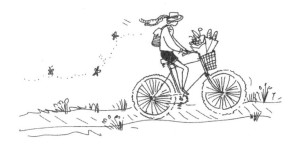

Whats the first thing to go when your daily schedule gets overburdened? For most people, it's exercise. But exercise helps you deal effectively with the physical and psychological demands of a hectic life. How do you find more time or use the time you have more wisely to get healthy, toned, and trim?

Exercise Is Essential

Break up your exercise routine into 10-minute segments and try to fit three to six segments into your day. The benefits are practically the same as if you were to do just one long routine.

Find a better way to commute to work. If possible, walk or ride your bicycle. If that isn't possible, park a mile or two away from work and hoof it to the office. If you take a train or bus, get off at the stop prior to your regular one. Your legs will soon reflect all this added mileage!

Find creative ways to integrate family time with exercise. If you have children, don't just be a bystander at the local playground; get up and climb the jungle gym with them, or run around the bases playing softball. Push a jogging stroller and give Junior a fun ride. Try bicycling, hiking, swimming, or just walking around the neighborhood with your family. Everyone will be healthier as a result.

Schedule your exercise time. Make it a priority and stick to it just as you would a scheduled doctor's or dentist's appointment.

Work out first thing in the morning. I find that if I get my exercise finished and out of the way, I don't have to try to fit it in at the end of the day when I'm usually tired and might be tempted to skip my workout altogether.

Combine work with exercise. Sound strange? I love to in-line skate and while I'm whizzing up and down my neighborhood streets, I carry a small tape recorder and make notes as I skate. My neighbors thought I was a bit strange at first, but they're used to me now. You can do this as you walk, also.

Make dinner while you exercise. If you enjoy one-pot dinners or main-course casseroles, pop one on the stove or into the oven and do your workout while it cooks. A Crock-Pot is a real blessing for busy people. It cooks long and slow so you can do other things while making dinner. As a bonus, exercising before you eat may take the edge off your appetite — and boost your metabolism, too.

Make exercise time *your* time. Remember, there's no better way to pamper yourself than by taking care of your health.

Health is something we do for ourselves, not something that is done to us; a journey rather than a destination; a dynamic, holistic, and purposeful way of living.

— Dr. Elliott Dacher

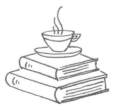

High-Energy Snacks

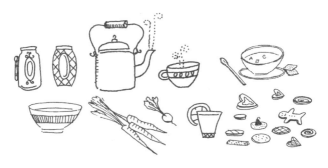

In the mood for a snack? Need fast food that will satisfy your cravings yet not be filled with empty calories and fat? Well, look no farther. Here are a few of my favorite delicious, guilt-free, quick snacks.

Need a Boost?

For a super-cooling summertime snack, nothing beats sweet, frozen, seedless grapes. They're a tasty, crunchy treat that's full of vitamins and minerals.

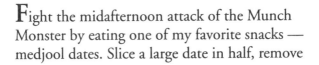

Fight the midafternoon attack of the Munch Monster by eating one of my favorite snacks — medjool dates. Slice a large date in half, remove

the pit, insert a raw pecan into each half, then
sprinkle with coconut flakes.

To organic plain yogurt or fortified soy yogurt,
add any or all of the following: ripe raspberries,
blackberries, sliced peaches, strawberries, kiwi,
papaya, almond slivers, raisins, granola. Stir well
and drizzle with honey or maple syrup, if desired.

For a high-protein snack, top melba toast or a rice
cake with peanut or sesame butter or cottage cheese.

Sweet-n-Nutty Snack Mix

*Convenient and portable, this mix is 100 percent better
for you than a candy bar or chips! You'll get approximately
3½ cups from this recipe.*

½ cup raw almonds
½ cup raw hazelnuts
½ cup dried, unsulfured, pitted cherries
½ cup large, unsulfured raisins
½ cup raw Brazil nuts
¼ cup lightly salted sunflower seeds, toasted
¼ cup lightly salted pumpkin seeds, toasted
¼ cup dried, unsulfured apricots, chopped
¼ cup carob or chocolate chips (optional)
Dash cinnamon or nutmeg (optional)

Place all ingredients in a plastic bag or food storage container and shake well. Keep tightly sealed in the refrigerator
unless consumed within two weeks; raw nuts become rancid
quicker than roasted ones. Consume a handful or so whenever the snacking mood strikes.

18

Harness the Power of Your Shower

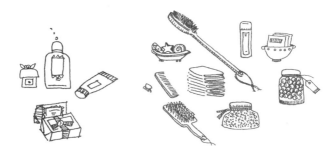

Turn your ordinary daily cleansing shower into a therapeutic spa. While a tub full of warm, sudsy, aromatic water conjures thoughts of relaxation, a shower can offer a wide array of body-pampering benefits simply by concentrating the flow of water onto specific body parts, enabling you to tackle problems such as sore muscles, headache, low energy, and lack-luster hair, to name a few.

Hydrotherapies

Increase Your Energy: Shower in water that's approximately body temperature for 2 to 3 minutes, then lower the temperature to very cool for about 15 to 30 seconds. Repeat this procedure twice more. Incidentally, this form of hydrotherapy has been used for centuries by many cultures to strengthen the immune system, thereby staving off colds and flus.

Hydrate Scaly Skin: For skin that resembles a desert reptile's, take a quickie shower for about 2 minutes in warm water. While your skin is still wet, slather on your favorite body oil, then pat dry.

Head Off a Headache: A handheld shower apparatus is best for this type of therapy. Turn on very warm water and aim the stream directly onto the aching area of your head for 5 minutes. Frequently, simply aiming the water onto the back of your head and neck will ease the pain. Some people find that alternating very warm and cold water every 30 seconds for 5 minutes works wonders, too.

Reduce Swelling: To reduce inflammation to an acute injury such as a burn, sprained ankle or wrist, or severely stubbed toe, aim a cold spray of water onto the affected part for 5 minutes, then off for 5 minutes, repeating a few times. Do this immediately after the injury occurs, then seek medical attention if necessary.

Relieve Sore Muscles: For muscles that are chronically sore or are sore from mere overexertion, but are not inflamed, aim a very warm water spray directly onto the muscle(s) for 5 minutes, then off for 5 minutes. Do this a few times.

Put an End to PMS Pain: To relieve lower-back pain occurring before and/or during menstruation, I find that a very warm stream of water concentrated on my lower back for a few minutes helps lessen the cramping and muscle tension. Follow with a rich moisturizer to avoid dry skin.

19

Condition Your Tresses

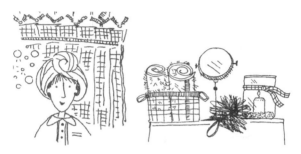

Most men and women today style their hair to some degree daily. Whether it's simply a quick blow-dry or a complex ritual of moussing, drying, using hot rollers, brushing, then topping it all off with hair spray, your hair takes a lot of abuse.

Consider, too, environmental stress. Sunshine, salt water, chlorine, cigarette smoke, pollution, and dry office air all take their toll — hair is not meant to take this kind of constant torture.

Restore Your Crowning Glory

The following recipes are quite simple to make and, with consistent use, will improve the condition of your hair and scalp.

To condition dry, brittle, damaged hair, mash a very ripe, large banana. Add a tablespoon each of heavy cream and honey and whisk together until smooth. Apply to dry hair from the roots to the ends, cover with a shower cap, and then wrap your head with a warm towel. Allow the mixture to remain on your hair for as long as possible — up to an hour. Rinse thoroughly with warm water, then shampoo as usual. If necessary, follow with a natural, detangling light conditioner.

Enhance the gloss of normal or dry hair with jojoba oil. Actually a plant wax, not an oil, this yellow substance closely resembles human sebum. It makes a superb scalp and hair conditioner. To 6 tablespoons of jojoba oil, add 1 teaspoon each of the following essential oils: rosemary, basil, lemon, and lavender. Store in a 4-ounce, dark glass bottle. Shake vigorously before each use. Use within one year for maximum potency. Apply 1 or 2 table-spoons to dry hair and scalp. There's no need to soak your hair; just make sure all the strands are coated thoroughly. Be sure to give your scalp a good 5-minute massage to stimulate circulation and encourage hair growth. Cover your head with a shower cap and wrap with a warm, damp towel for up to an hour. Shampoo and follow with a good, light detangling conditioner if necessary. This treatment may be used weekly.

Rinse, rinse, rinse. If smooth and silky hair is your aim, proper rinsing is crucial. Even the best conditioners will leave your hair drab and dull if not rinsed out completely.

Tressonaise

Smooth your mane with this recipe for homemade mayonnaise filled with hair-healthy conditioning ingredients that will add shine and softness.

    I whole egg plus I yolk (room temperature)
  I½ tablespoons lemon juice
    I cup unrefined olive, avocado, or sesame oil

1. Break the eggs into the blender, add lemon juice, and blend on medium for about 5 seconds. Remove the center plastic stopper from the cover, turn the blender back on, and begin to drizzle the oil in a slow, steady stream until all the oil is used. The mayonnaise should now be nice and thick.

2. Scrape out the mayonnaise using a long, flexible spatula and store in a covered, glass container in the refrigerator. This recipe makes one treatment for long hair, two treatments for shoulder-length hair, or three treatments for short hair.

3. To dry hair, apply enough mayonnaise to cover the damaged parts. If you have an oily scalp but dry, frizzy, damaged ends, then treat only the lower portion of your hair. Cover your hair with a shower cap or plastic bag, then wrap with a warm towel. Allow to remain on your hair for up to an hour, then shampoo once or twice to remove all traces of oil. Follow with your usual conditioner if you need to detangle. You may use once a week, if desired.

20

Take the Sting Out of Sunburn

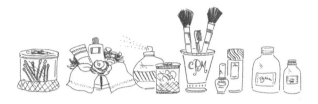

It happens every spring: One of those unseasonably warm days comes along to tease and tantalize and make you throw caution to the wind. You decide to toss on your skimpiest bathing suit, bare your sun-starved skin to the warm air, and soak up a few rays. A few hours later, you wake up from dreamland. You run inside, look in the mirror, and uh-oh, you look like a lobster — and it hurts!

It's essential to rehydrate your skin immediately following a burn to restore pH balance and soothe the tender, injured tissue.

Soothe That Sunburn

Refrigerate your creams and lotions during hot weather for a skin-chilling, sunburn-soothing treat!

Add 2 cups of apple cider vinegar to cool bath-water. Soak for 10 to 20 minutes.

Spray a chilled German chamomile or lavender aromatic hydrosol directly onto the sunburned area to reduce redness and inflammation.

Spread yogurt or sour cream on itchy, burning skin for quick, super-cool relief.

Apply cold, strong, black tea directly to sunburn with soaked cotton pads. Use several times per day.

Aloe After-Sun Relief Spray

For skin that's hot, itchy, red, tender, and possibly blistered, reduce the temperature by taking a cold bath or shower. Pat your skin dry, then generously spray on this formula. Store the spray in the refrigerator for up to six months.

      1 cup aloe vera juice (*not* gel)
     20 drops essential oil of lavender
     20 drops essential oil of carrot seed
     10 drops essential oil of calendula
      5 drops essential oil of peppermint or rosemary
         (optional, for cooling effect)

1. Place all ingredients in an 8-ounce, dark glass spray bottle and shake well. Spray on sensitive burned skin as often as necessary to help hydrate, soothe, and protect.

2. Follow the spray treatment with a good, thick, natural moisturizer to help restore pliability to your dried-out skin. Pat, don't rub or massage, into the sunburned skin

21

Anti-aging
Secrets

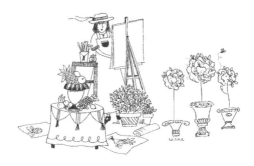

The search for the ever-elusive Fountain of Youth is still going strong. This is evidenced by the scores of commercials advertising the sale of anti-wrinkle creams, skin-lightening creams, energy-boosting nutrition supplements, and memory-enhancing herbal products, not to mention the increasing popularity of plastic surgery.

The way I see it, true youthfulness can't be purchased in a bottle or from a doctor. But the attributes of youth — smooth skin, an alert mind, an active, limber body — can be prolonged into old age by adhering to a youthful lifestyle and using common sense.

Maintain a Youthful Lifestyle

The old adage, "Early to bed, early to rise, makes you healthy, wealthy, and wise," still rings true today. Getting plenty of quality, sound sleep allows your body to rest, recharge, repair, and replenish so you'll be rarin' to go the next day.

Stimulate your brain. Don't allow yourself to become bored with life. Pick up a new hobby, find a new challenge, go back to school, read more. You *can* teach an old "dog" new tricks!

Become a "people person." Reach out and try to help someone every day.

Slow down; pace yourself. Quit scurrying around like a squirrel preparing its nest for winter. You can't enjoy life if you run through it at breakneck speed.

Get a pet. Studies show that pet owners live healthier, happier, less stressful lives.

Hydrate your skin. Dry skin ages prematurely, exhibiting lines and wrinkles long before Mother Nature intended. Apply a good moisturizing lotion each morning and evening. Don't forget to consume eight glasses of pure water daily, too!

Wear sunscreen. Nothing ages your skin faster than exposure to the sun's rays. Sun damage is cumulative. That golden tan of youth will eventually produce unwelcome wrinkles, uneven pigmentation, age spots, and potentially skin cancer in your middle and later years.

Eat fresh, whole, unprocessed foods. Avoid empty-calorie, junky, chemical-laden foods. They do nothing but satisfy a temporary craving. Real food satisfies your soul and truly nourishes your body.

Exercise daily. Use it or lose it! A sedentary lifestyle contributes to obesity, cardiovascular problems, stiff joints, lackluster skin and hair, and low energy — all signs of old age.

Keep a positive attitude. Negativity not only affects your mood, your job performance, your physical appearance, and your health in general, but affects the people around you as well. No one wants to be around a person with low self-esteem.

Simplify your life. It's not the material things in life that bring true happiness, it's friends, family, good food, pets, and time spent doing things you most enjoy.

22

Stay Cool & Dry

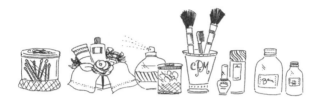

Natural body and foot powders are a chemical-free way to fight odor and perspiration. You can easily make your own customized body powders that will keep you cool and dry all day long.

Herbal Body & Foot Powders

Some excellent base-powder choices to use alone or in combination include cornstarch, rice flour, arrowroot, French clay, white cosmetic clay, powdered calendula flowers, and powdered chamomile flowers. Customize your powder by adding your favorite essential oils or powdered flowers. Powders are simple to formulate and are great gifts.

My favorite mixture is 1 part cornstarch, 1 part arrowroot, and 1 part powdered calendula flow-

ers. This mixture makes for a very light powder
— perfect for infants.

To keep your feet cool, dry, and odor-free, try
this blend: Combine ½ cup of baking soda,
2 tablespoons of zinc oxide powder, 2 tablespoons
of white cosmetic clay, ½ cup of arrowroot, and
1 teaspoon of essential oil of orange, geranium, or
peppermint. If you have athlete's foot or particularly odoriferous feet, substitute ½ teaspoon each
of essential oil of tea tree and thyme. To make,
follow the directions in the recipe below. Sprinkle
into your shoes and socks once or twice daily.

For those with allergies, a powder made from
100 percent arrowroot powder, cornstarch, or
white cosmetic clay will generally be irritation-free.

Lavender Powder

*This is a delightfully soft, silky body powder. The recipe
makes about 1⅛ cups.*

- ½ cup white cosmetic clay, arrowroot, or cornstarch
- ¼ cup powdered lavender flowers
- ¼ cup powdered rose petals
- 1 tablespoon zinc oxide powder
- ½ teaspoon essential oil of lavender
- 10 drops essential oil of rose (optional)

Mix the dry ingredients in a large bowl or food processor.
Add the essential oils a few drops at a time and thoroughly
incorporate into the powder. Store this in a special shaker
container or recycled spice jar. Use within one year.

23

Cultivate Some
ZZZZZZZZZS

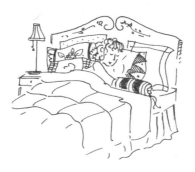

Has your get-up-and-go got up and gone? Suffering from brain fog? Too much on your mind to relax? Feeling constantly cranky? Insomnia a problem lately? Sleep deprivation takes its toll on both your face and body in a hurry. To look and feel your absolute best, you need to get approximately seven to nine hours of deeply restful, quality sleep each night.

"Perchance to Dream..."

Flannel sheets are an insomniac's best friend! Year-round, I sleep between thick, 6-ounce flannels that feel like light, soft, velvety blankets of fluffy cotton. During hot summer weather, forgo the usual thin blanket and substitute the top flannel sheet as your cover.

Get plenty of vigorous exercise early in the day so you'll be naturally tired come bedtime. Exercise performed too close to retiring can be too stimulating for some people.

Sip a cup of hot catnip, chamomile, or raspberry leaf herbal tea. Hot, mineral-rich vegetable broth, cow's milk, and calcium-fortified soy or rice milk are also good. Drink it an hour prior to bedtime or you'll wake up needing to visit the lavatory.

Don't go to bed on a full stomach. Digestion takes lots of energy and will keep you awake.

Go to bed at the same time every night. Once your body gets used to a routine, it will naturally want to fall asleep at that time.

Put a drop or two of soothing essential oil of lavender or Roman chamomile on your pillow.

Avoid caffeinated products such as certain brands of pain relievers, diet pills, and the usual culprits — coffee, cola drinks, chocolate, and black tea. Not only does caffeine keep you awake, but it also makes for more restless sleep and acts as a diuretic, causing you to make more trips to the bathroom.

Install light-blocking curtains or shades. These will help you stay asleep.

Purchase a device that drowns out disturbing noises and produces sleep-inducing sounds such as ocean waves lapping the shore, a gently babbling brook, or wind in the trees.

There must be stillness for the spirit to enter.

— Anonymous

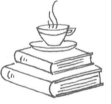

Sleepytime Balm

So simple to make, yet so effective. Gentle enough to safely pacify even the most irritable, restless infant.

- ¼ cup all-vegetable shortening (room temperature)
- 10 drops essential oil of orange
- 2 drops essential oil of ylang-ylang
- 1 drop essential oil of vanilla (optional)

Combine all ingredients in a small bowl and whip together using a small spatula or whisk. Apply a dab of balm to your temples after cleansing your face and just prior to bedtime. Use daily, if desired. Store in a 2-ounce plastic or glass jar in a dry, cool place for up to three or four months.

Fortify Yourself against Cold & Flu

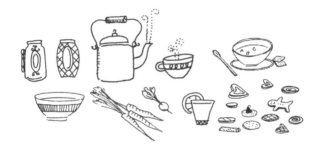

"Feed a fever, starve a cold." Or is it "Feed a cold, starve a fever"? All I know is that when I'm achy, stuffy, and miserable, I want relief and I want it fast!

Commercial flu and cold medications always leave me feeling woozy or severely parch my sinuses and throat. They offer nothing in the way of health benefits, only temporary symptom relief.

After years of experimentation, I've finally hit upon two tried-and-true formulas that are guaranteed to return you to the land of the living in no time at all. They're nutritious and delicious ways to help your body heal itself without leaving you feeling like a blob!

Zesty Cider

A spicy, warming, tasty, natural antibiotic. This cider tastes good as a zippy salad dressing, too! Try to use organic ingredients. This recipe makes approximately 1½ quarts.

50 cloves garlic (not elephant garlic), minced

3 tablespoons dried or 6 tablespoons fresh echinacea root, grated or chopped

¾ cup fresh horseradish root, grated

½ cup fresh gingerroot, peeled and sliced

3 medium-size white onions, diced

I teaspoon cayenne pepper powder or 3 fresh habañero peppers, diced and seeded

Honey to sweeten, if desired

2 quarts raw apple cider vinegar

1. Place all ingredients in a 2-quart widemouthed jar. Fill to the top with vinegar. Cover the top of the jar with plastic wrap, then screw on the lid.

2. Refrigerate for six weeks so the flavor can develop and soften. Shake daily. There's no need to strain and bottle unless you want to. I think the flavor keeps getting better and bolder the longer the formula is allowed to steep.

3. At the first sign of a cold or flu, take 2 tablespoons of Zesty Cider with a warm water chaser. Rinse your mouth out well after swallowing the cider. Repeat once or twice daily for the duration of the illness. You should feel your sinus and bronchial passages quickly open and breathing become easier.

4. For a sore throat, gargle with the Zesty Cider straight for 60 seconds, spit, then rinse out your mouth. You should feel immediate relief.

Southwestern Chicken-Vegetable Soup

A very warming, spicy soup that serves up immune-boosting nutrition and opens sinus and bronchial passages, allowing for freer breathing. Try to use organic ingredients. This soup freezes well, and the recipe makes approximately 15 cups.

     1 medium-size white onion, diced
    20 cloves garlic (not elephant garlic), minced
     2 celery stalks, sliced very thin
     2 tablespoons extra-virgin olive oil
     8 cups homemade chicken stock
     3 carrots, sliced very thin or cubed
     2 medium-size potatoes, cubed
     1 tablespoon fresh lemon juice
    ½ teaspoon cayenne pepper powder or 1 habañero
        pepper, diced and seeded
     1 tablespoon fresh parsley, minced
     2 teaspoons fresh cilantro, minced
     1 bay leaf
        Salt, pepper, oregano, savory, rosemary, or thyme
        to taste

In a 4-quart stock pot, sauté the onion, garlic, and celery in olive oil until transparent. Add the remaining ingredients and bring to a boil. Reduce the heat, and then cover and simmer for an hour. Eat a bowl whenever you feel the need for feasting and fortification.

25

Make Your Own Bath & Massage Oils

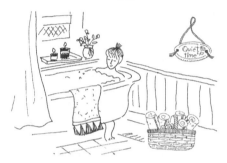

Bath and massage oils are very easy to make at home. You simply need a base oil and any essential oil you desire. I like to use jojoba oil as my base because it does not need refrigeration and will not go rancid. Grapeseed, apricot kernel, and hazelnut oils also make great base oils because they are very light, but they must be refrigerated.

Soften and Scent Your Skin

Uplifting, Energizing Oil: Combine 1 tablespoon of jojoba oil with 2 drops each of essential oils of peppermint, rosemary, and eucalyptus. Add to your bath while the tap is running. For a deodorizing foot treatment, have a friend massage your clean, tired feet with the oil for 15 minutes. Then put on socks, and go to bed.

Exotic Oil: This formula conditions dry skin and leaves a sensual, musky fragrance. Mix together ¾ cup jojoba oil with ¼ teaspoon each of these essential oils: sandalwood, patchouli, vetiver. Then add ¼ teaspoon of synthetic musk oil (optional). Store away from heat and light in a tightly sealed, 8-ounce, dark glass bottle. To use, add 2 teaspoons of oil to the bath while the tub is filling. For massage, use ½ teaspoon of essential oil blend to ½ cup of jojoba oil. For an exotic perfume, mix the essential oils only and bottle.

Nourishing Oil

This vitamin- and mineral-rich formula is good for all skin types, especially normal and dry. Excellent for dry, ragged cuticles, too.

- 1 tablespoon almond oil
- 1 tablespoon extra-virgin olive oil
- 1 tablespoon avocado oil
- 1 tablespoon jojoba oil
- 1 tablespoon apricot kernel oil
- 1 tablespoon hazelnut oil
- 1,200 international units (IUs) vitamin E oil (d-alpha tocopherol)

Combine all ingredients in an 8-ounce glass or plastic bottle. Tightly cap and shake vigorously. Store in the refrigerator for up to a year. For your bath, add 2 teaspoons to running water. For massage, use directly on your skin as needed.

26

Pamper Those Peepers

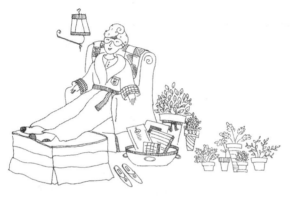

I t's said that the eyes are the windows to the soul. But if you look at a computer screen all day, party all night, spend time around smokers or in dry office air, have allergies, or forget to remove your mascara, your "windows" are going to look puffy, bloodshot, or irritated, or they'll have dark circles beneath them. They may even sting and tear.

Add Sparkle to Your Eyes

Your eyes are your most expressive features — do your best to pamper them. Follow these suggestions to soothe, brighten, and refresh red and weary eyes.

Pep up your pretty peepers with plenty of sound sleep — one of the best beautifiers there is!

Swollen eyes and dark circles can sometimes be the result of toxin buildup in the body, as well as dehydration. When the body is dehydrated, the kidneys try to retain water, which results in puffiness. Drink plenty of water daily in order to flush toxins and excess sodium from your body. The more water you drink, the less you will retain.

For swollen eyelids, dip cotton balls or cosmetic squares into icy-cold whole milk or cream. Lie down, and apply soaked cotton to your eyelids. Leave on for 5 to 10 minutes. The high fat content of either liquid provides a moisturizing treatment for the delicate, thin skin around your eyes.

Tune out. Don't be a TV addict. The glare from the screen is not good for your eyes. Besides, you can spend your time more wisely.

See your way clear by eliminating sore, dry, red, irritated eyes. My favorite treatment is to keep handy a bottle of lavender aromatic hydrosol and spritz my face and eyes with it as often as necessary. The liquid is so pure and gentle that I can spray it directly into my opened eyes. I find it extremely soothing. German chamomile and rose hydrosol work equally well.

Apply a chilled, water-based lotion or gel around the eye area once a day after cleansing to moisturize the delicate skin. A cucumber-based product is a good choice.

A daily application of sunscreen to the skin on and around your eyes is essential if you want to prevent sun damage and the formation of dark circles. Choose a product specifically designed to be used on the face.

Add 2 or 3 drops of essential oil of calendula to a small jar of chilled herbal eye cream. The resulting bright orange cream will help offset the blue color of dark circles, and the calendula essential oil is guaranteed to restore and soothe tired eyes, leaving them revived and refreshed.

Out of eye makeup remover? Apply a dab of all-vegetable shortening to the eye area and gently rub over your lashes. It will dissolve even the most stubborn waterproof mascara and eyeliner. Makes a great impromptu moisturizer for dry patches of eczema and psoriasis, too!

Give Yourself a Pedicure

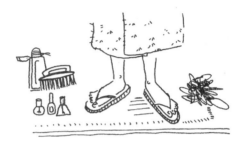

What's the next best thing to a full-body massage? A professional pedicure. Take my word for it, the procedure is incredibly relaxing. If you can't fit a visit to your local nail technician into your budget or schedule, then you'll just have to pamper those tootsies yourself. A do-it-yourself pedicure will leave your feet fresh and supple, and you'll be in a better frame of mind, guaranteed!

Feet First

Set aside about an hour one evening per week to treat your feet. Surround yourself with all of the necessary supplies so you don't have to keep getting up and dripping water all over the house. Then follow these steps for smoother, more beautiful feet.

Step 1: The feet are one of the most receptive parts of the body, and a footbath is often just as relaxing or stimulating as a full-body bath. To your foot tub, add enough hot or cold water or herbal tea of your choice to cover your ankles, then a few drops of tea tree essential oil or a squirt of liquid soap or shower gel. Swish together. Soak your feet for 5 to 10 minutes to cleanse and soften calluses. Use this time to scrub your dirty toenails and soles using a toenail brush.

Step 2: After soaking, gently remove calluses with a pediwand, rasp, or stone. File down any corns with an emery board or diamond file.

Step 3: Dry your feet and legs when finished and remove any old, chipped nail polish using an oily, nonacetone nail polish remover.

Step 4: Time to exfoliate. Apply a mixture of 1 tablespoon each of salt and extra-virgin olive oil, plus 5 drops essential oil of peppermint to your feet and lower legs. Massage in circular motions concentrating on your heels, ankles, and any particularly rough, thickened areas. It will scrub off any leftover rough skin, and it feels and smells fantastic, too! Rinse your feet and legs. Dry with a coarse towel.

Step 5: Coax back cuticles with an orange stick and trim any that are ragged. Trim toenails straight across, rather than rounded at the corners, so that the white free edge is almost even with the top of the toe. File your toenails to smooth any jagged edges.

Step 6: Apply foot lotion, oil, or cream and massage in thoroughly for 2 or 3 minutes on each foot.

Step 7: If you're polishing your toenails, apply nail polish remover now to remove all traces of lotion or cream. Dry the nails. Now slick on a base coat, then two coats of your favorite color, followed by a top coat — allow each coat to dry in between. There's nothing like 10 freshly painted, glossy, perfectly pedicured toes to pick you up and make you feel pretty!

Step 8: After your polish dries, apply your favorite powder to your legs and feet, using a large puff or fluff brush to scent and prevent perspiration from taking a foothold.

28

Flower Power

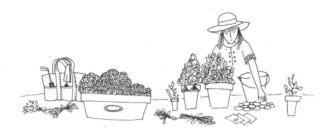

The calendula flower, or pot marigold, is one flower you should familiarize yourself with. It's a beautiful, cheery, daisylike plant that is easy to grow in full sun and average soil; it can withstand heat, cold, drought, and even some dampness. This lovely, hardy flower has been used for centuries to gently and effectively heal many ills.

Rejuvenate and Heal

To heal minor cuts, scrapes, bee stings, and burns, apply calendula infused oil (see the recipe opposite) directly to the irritation.

For hard-to-heal dry, cracked skin, try calendula salve. For an instant salve, combine ¼ cup of room-temperature all-vegetable shortening with 20 drops essential oil of calendula. Stir well. Massage into affected parts as often as desired. This recipe also makes a soothing, gentle cream for diaper rash and ragged cuticles.

For an earache, place a few drops of warm calendula infused oil into each ear, plug with cotton balls, and leave overnight.

To brighten a salad, add fresh calendula blossoms along with violets and nasturtiums for a variety of tastes, textures, and colors.

Calendula Blossom Oil

You'll make about 4 cups of a potent healing oil that can be used as a salve base, massage oil, or bath oil. You can also use it in any healing formula calling for oil.

> 4–5 cups calendula blossoms, wilted for 24 hours in well-ventilated shade
> Extra-virgin olive oil

1. Put the calendula blossoms in a 3-quart pot and pour in enough olive oil to cover by 2 inches. Turn the burner on low. Heat the mixture to just below a simmer, and let it steep for 5 to 10 hours, uncovered. Check on it every hour or so to make sure the oil isn't simmering.

2. Remove from the heat after the oil smells herby and has attained a rich, golden-orange color. Cool, strain, bottle, label, and refrigerate. This oil will keep for six months to a year if refrigerated. Use within 60 days if not refrigerated.

29

Professional Pampering Tips

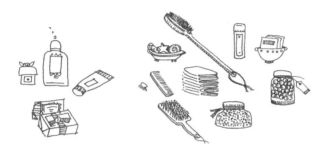

S elf-pampering is a wonderful way to address your emotional, physical, and spiritual needs, but sometimes it just plain feels better to put yourself into the hands of a professional. Here are some tips for a great pampering experience.

Day Spa Specialties

N ever had a full-body massage before? Then try a mini massage. Many day spas offer low-fee or even complimentary mini massages for your back, shoulders, or feet to entice prospective customers to sign up for a full treatment.

Next time you visit your hairstylist or barber, ask the shampoo technician to spend extra time performing a scalp massage. The tension will simply drain from your head. Make sure to tip him or her appropriately for a job well done.

Try an energy-balancing treatment such as reiki or polarity therapy. These noninvasive techniques can be used to facilitate all types of healing.

A spa manicure or pedicure is a change of pace from the usual variety. These can include a sea salt soak, a mud or paraffin mask, a full hand-and-foot reflexology treatment, followed by a softening peppermint cream massage. Ahhhh...

If you happen to be visiting a resort or hotel that offers mud baths, sign up! Warm, gooey, mineral-rich mud removes toxins from the skin and tones and tightens the pores. It's terrific for easing muscular and joint pain, too.

To soften, hydrate, and exfoliate your body, try a seaweed or herbal body wrap. These treatments are especially beneficial after a summer vacation in which your skin has been overexposed.

30

Brighten Your Home with Flowering Plants

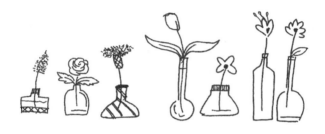

I was born with a green thumb, inherited from my grandmother. It's a true blessing! Everything I touch seems to explode with bountiful growth and flowers. But fear not: Even if you're a certified "brown thumb," you can add brilliance, beauty, and fragrance to your home by cultivating these easy-to-grow varieties of plants.

The Power of Flowers

Nothing is prettier and more cheery than a room full of colorful flowering plants. Why not fill your home with blooms? One of the easiest plants to grow is the Christmas cactus. If you have several sunny windows in your home, buy a few plants in red, white, salmon, pale pink, fuchsia, and the rare golden-orange (if you can find it). Plant them in clay pots, and you'll enjoy bountiful blooms from Thanksgiving through Christmas and possibly again around Easter. These plants require minimal care, and like to be potbound.

Try your hand at forcing flowering bulbs — causing bulbs to bloom out of season so that they bloom inside your home in the dead of winter. In the fall, visit your local nursery and pick up 5 to 10 hyacinth, paperwhite, daffodil, or tulip bulbs, a relatively shallow pot especially for forcing bulbs, and a small bag of white gravel, shells, or marbles. Pour a layer of your chosen material about an inch deep in the bottom of the pot; insert your bulbs root-side down into the gravel, shells, or marbles; then pour enough material around the bulbs to reach about midbulb height. Fertilize with a liquid flowering-plant fertilizer and keep the base of the bulbs moist, not swimming in water, until flowering is complete. Set the pot in a bright, sunny window and wait for blooming time.

If you receive a potted amaryllis bulb for Christmas, be sure to save it, pot and all, after it has finished blooming. Keep it indoors, barely moist, until nighttime temperatures drop no lower than 40° F, and then set it on your patio or steps in partial sun for the remainder of the year. About early November, cut off all growth down to bulb-tip level, give it a good drink of liquid fertilizer, and put it in a sunny window. In a few months you'll have another round of blossoms, possibly more than the year before. Amaryllis bulbs grow larger each year, and the number of stems and blossoms increases as each bulb ages. These are large, showy flowers, growing about 1 to 2 feet tall, and available in a rainbow of colors.

Love the look of orchids, but afraid they might be hard to grow? Consult your local nursery about the how-tos of orchid growing and soon you'll have these delicate yet long-blooming beauties throughout your home. They're actually quite easy to grow provided your home temperature doesn't drop below 55° F in the winter. The common phalaenopsis orchid blooms for about four months, comes in a variety of colors and sizes, and is simply glorious!

Buy a book on flowering houseplants and read up on proper care instructions for your newly acquired beauties. Some of my plants are so big now that I can't get them out of the house; they've outgrown the door width! Learn how, when, and with what to fertilize your plants, how much water and light they need, and when to transplant them for optimum health and growth.

31

Have a Honey of a Day

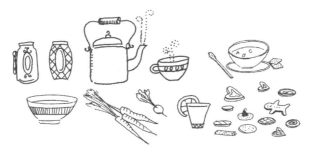

Honey — that sweet, thick, golden syrup produced by thousands of honeybees — not only tastes great on food but, as the Native Americans discovered, can also help heal myriad ailments, nourish your body, and soften your skin. Who would have thought that an everyday food could have so many uses?

Life Is Sweet

Cut your finger or scrape your knee? Put a few drops of honey on the affected area. Honey has been proven to be just as effective in most cases as standard topical antibacterial ointments and helps keep the cut or abrasion sterile and the surrounding skin soft so scarring is minimized.

Suffering from dry, finely lined skin? Try a "honey tap" facial. Moisten the skin, then apply a very thin layer of honey onto your face and neck (make sure to put your hair up first or things could get sticky) by tapping your honey-laden fingertips over your skin. The tapping revs up circulation, and the honey acts as a humectant to draw moisture to your skin. Lie down for about 15 minutes, then rinse with warm water. Your skin should be rosy, warm, moist, and glowing.

For nursing mothers, try massaging a dab of honey on dry, cracked, sore nipples. This is reported to soften the skin and aid in healing. Just make sure to rinse off the honey before nursing again, as infants under 12 months of age should not consume honey.

HEALING HONEY TIP

Use only unprocessed honey for topical use. It's available from health-food stores or from an apiary. It's not the same as the usual grocery-store varieties, which have been heated and filtered, rendering the beneficial enzymes and nutrients cooked and lifeless.

Soothe a sore throat by gargling with a cup of warm sage-honey tea. To a cup of boiling water, add 1 teaspoon dried sage. Steep for 5 minutes, and then strain. Add 1 tablespoon honey and stir. Gargle for 60 seconds as often as needed throughout the day; spit out the liquid. Rinse your mouth with water after each use so the natural sugars don't remain on your teeth.

Sweet Energy

This pick-me-up drink is chock-full of potassium, a natural energizer, in addition to B vitamins, fructose, glucose, and trace minerals. It is quite refreshing and invigorating, and can be drunk twice daily, especially when you're tired, achy, or suffering from stiff joints. This formula is reported to relieve the pain and inflammation of arthritis if consumed daily.

> 2 teaspoons raw, unheated, unfiltered apple cider vinegar (available in health-food stores)
> 1 teaspoon raw honey
> 6–8 ounces water

Stir ingredients thoroughly in a glass and drink on an empty stomach. You can also use this liquid as a facial splash for sunburned, dehydrated skin.

32

Keep Your Skin in Super Shape

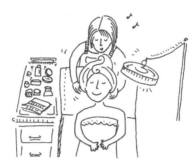

Professional estheticians (skin-care special-
ists) agree that there are certain basic proce-
dures and rituals you must follow to ensure
a lifetime of beautiful skin. Caring for your skin
shouldn't be a chore, nor should it cost a fortune.
Follow these simple tips recommended by my
fellow esthetician friends for skin that is plump,
soft, rosy, and glowing with vitality.

Esthetic Essentials

Try to have a professional facial at least twice a year.

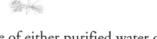

Keep a mister bottle of either purified water or
herbal aromatic hydrosol (available in health-food

stores) handy at all times to refresh and hydrate your skin whenever you start to feel dry. This is especially important if you're a frequent flier.

Drink, drink, drink ... at least eight glasses of purified water every day.

Use sunscreen daily with a sun protection factor (SPF) of at least 15.

Cleanse, tone, and moisturize twice a day with products specifically created for your skin type. As you get older, reevaluate your skin type. Everything changes with age!

Eat a healthy diet and get plenty of outdoor exercise.

Learn to manage the stress in your life. Stress wreaks havoc on even the most beautiful skin.

Not only does beauty fade, but it leaves a record upon the face as to what became of it.

— Elbert Hubbard

33

Strengthen Your Fingernails

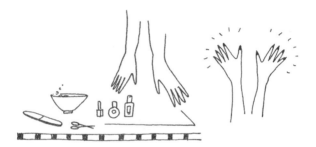

Beautiful, strong fingernails are generally a sign of good health and good habits. Your fingernails can become weak and brittle for a variety of reasons, such as lack of moisture, exposure to the elements or harsh household cleansers, or simply lack of proper care. See Nourish Your Nails, page 112, for more tips.

No-Nonsense Nail Care

Massage cuticles with a good, thick moisturizer or a dab of castor oil or vitamin E before bedtime.

Don't use your fingernails as tools. Instead, use a paper clip, screwdriver, or knife tip to pry something open or scrape off old candle wax or tape.

Don't cut your cuticles. Healthy cuticles contribute to healthy nails. Instead, gently push back oiled or moisturized cuticles with an orange stick wrapped with a small piece of flannel or soft cloth.

File your nails in one direction only; don't saw back and forth. Professional manicurists recommend using a diamond-dust or ceramic file to shape nails to a nice blunt oval.

Steer clear of fake nails. Research has shown that the chemical ingredients used for artificial nails and glue weaken the natural nail. There is also the potential for harmful fungus and bacteria accumulation.

Castor Oil Soak

This formula is good for dry, brittle, weak nails and cuticles. It takes just minutes to make and doubles as a terrific massage oil for dry hands.

    4–5 tablespoons castor oil
    10 drops essential oil of carrot seed or frankincense
    Contents of a small vitamin E capsule

In a small bowl, combine the oils. Soak clean fingertips for 5 to 10 minutes. Using a soft cloth, push back your cuticles and lightly buff your nails. You can use the same mixture for three treatments if it's kept covered and refrigerated.

34

Freshen Your Breath

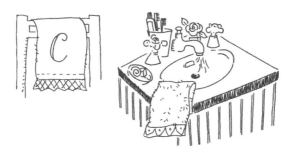

Most commercial mouthwashes only serve to temporarily mask mouth odors, and contain artificial dyes, synthetic flavors, and harsh chemicals. Don't just cover up the odor, get rid of it by eliminating the cause of the problem.

No Offense!

For an antiseptic mouthwash and gargle, add 3 or 4 drops of essential oil of clove to 4 ounces of water. Swish in your mouth and gargle.

For breath that's tingly and spicy-sweet, suck on a dried clove or two.

Charcoal is a time-tested ingredient used to absorb poisons from the stomach, relieve gas pains, help treat diarrhea, and act as a breath purifier. Buy charcoal capsules; follow label directions.

Pyorrhea, or infected gums, can produce an unpleasant taste and odor in the mouth and should be seen by a dentist. In conjunction with your dentist's recommendations, dip a cotton swab into myrrh tincture and apply directly to sore gums and loose teeth.

Fight bad breath, clean your teeth, and stimulate your gums at the same time by using dental floss impregnated with essential oil of tea tree (available in better health-food stores). It is highly antibacterial and helps neutralize strong mouth odor.

After eating an especially garlicky meal, thoroughly chew a sprig of parsley and drink a cup of strong peppermint tea. Both herbs freshen your breath and also act as digestive aids.

For a super-effective antibacterial breath spray, combine ¼ cup each of distilled water and vodka, plus 5 drops each of essential oils of clove, anise, cinnamon, and orange. Store in a 4-ounce, dark glass bottle with a mister top. Shake before each use.

35

Protect Your Skin from the Sun

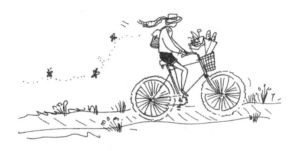

L ight to moderate exposure to the sun makes us feel good, helps the body manufacture vitamin D, gives us energy, and leaves a rosy-golden glow upon the skin. On the flipside, overexposure dries our skin, causing wrinkles, blotchiness, and premature aging. Sun protection is a hot topic these days.

Sun-Savvy Tips

In my opinion, 10 to 20 minutes of sun exposure several days a week, sans sunscreen, before 10:30 A.M. or after 4:30 P.M., is good for your physical health as well as your emotional well-being. However, if you are going to be in the sun for a longer period of time, by all means apply a sunscreen with an SPF of at least 15. Make sure the label indicates that the product provides UVA and UVB broad-spectrum protection.

Sensitive to chemical sunscreens? Try the titanium-dioxide-based products. Titanium dioxide is a natural mineral that acts as a physical block to UVA and UVB rays.

Remember the thick white stuff lifeguards used to put on their noses? That old standby, white zinc oxide cream, is still available, but now it's also offered in colors, which children really love. This cream totally blocks the sun. If you need every bit of protection possible, use zinc oxide cream on sunburn-prone areas such as your lips (be careful not to ingest), nose, ears, and shoulders.

There is no safe tan! Applying a topical vitamin C cream with a sunblock increases its effectiveness against skin damage, dehydration, and wrinkles.

The sun parches your skin, sucking it dry, so try to find a moisturizing sunscreen or apply your sunscreen first, allow it to dry, then apply a moisturizer on top of it.

PAYING A HIGH PRICE

In the July 1998 issue of *Elle* magazine, dermatologist Dr. Patricia Wexler stated, "More than 90 percent of the damage we see in aging is due to sun exposure. The sun damage you get today will show up twenty years later in terms of wrinkles, large pores, loss of elasticity, uneven pigmentation, precancerous cells, age spots, and skin cancer .... It's never too late to start with sunblock, but you shouldn't keep stalling."

Sunscreen Body Oil

This formula is good for normal and dry skin, medium or dark skin, or when minimal to moderate sunscreen protection is desired. **Caution:** *If you are fair skinned, you will likely need more protection. This recipe makes approximately 1⅛ cups of body oil.*

- ¼ cup anhydrous lanolin
- ¼ cup unrefined sesame oil
- 4 teaspoons vitamin E oil
- ¼ cup jojoba oil
- ⅓ cup aloe vera juice (*not* gel)
- 15 drops essential oil of bitter almond or patchouli, or 2–3 drops coconut fragrance oil

Combine all ingredients in one or two plastic squeeze bottles. Shake thoroughly before application. Reapply after swimming. Between uses, store the bottle(s) in the refrigerator. Use unrefrigerated oil within three weeks or discard.

36

If It Feels Good, Do It

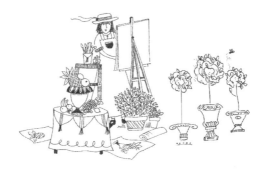

When you were a child, did you run barefoot in the newly mown lawn just because it felt cool and wet and because you liked having green feet? Did you play in a warm summer rain shower just because it smelled fresh and felt so good on your hot skin? Did you go down to the local creek and stomp around in the gooey mud and let it squish between your toes just because it was there?

As adults, many of us have gotten stodgy and set in our ways. We've forgotten that life can actually be fun and silly and full of feel-good things. For once, just try being a child again. Do something out of the ordinary — just because you can!

What Should I Do?

Sing all day long — children do.

Skip everywhere you go. Feel like a child all over again.

Give your feet a vacation. If possible, don't wear shoes for a week, or just wear simple rubber flip-flops.

Take a walk in the rain and don't worry about what the neighbors will think when they see your hair dripping wet. As an added bonus, your hair will feel as soft as cat fur when it dries, and be nicely conditioned, too.

Take a hike in the woods when it's snowing. Notice how fresh and clean the air smells and how quiet and still it is.

How lush and lusty the grass looks! How green!

— **William Shakespeare**

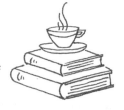

Have a big glass of chocolate cow's milk or soy milk with breakfast. How long has it been since you enjoyed this yummy drink?

Buy a butterfly net and gently catch, identify, and release these delicate, beautiful creatures.

Collect colorful seashells on the beach. Fill an inexpensive, clear glass lamp base with the shells. You'll be reminded of your fun day at the beach every time you turn on that lamp.

If you have a garden, forgo the shoes for one day and feel the warm, soft earth caress your feet. If a rain shower happens to pass over, keep gardening. Enjoy the different scents, textures of the leaves, and insect life around you. It's amazing how vibrant you feel while communing this closely with Mother Nature.

If you have a dog or are friendly with a neighbor's dog, don't just simply pat him on the head; bend down and give him a bear hug. Ever notice what children do when they see a big, friendly dog? If they're not afraid of animals, they'll run right up to him and give him a great big full-body hug. He'll love the attention and so will you, in return.

37

Here's Zucchini on Your Face!

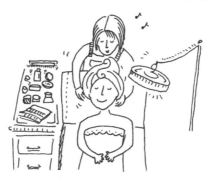

And mint, and sage, and raspberries, and apples. Did you know that these common foods can do double duty by nourishing your insides and beautifying your outsides?

Beauty from Your Garden

Try these blends for five days of quick, fresh-picked skin-pampering treatments.

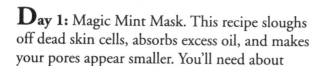

Day 1: Magic Mint Mask. This recipe sloughs off dead skin cells, absorbs excess oil, and makes your pores appear smaller. You'll need about

10 large peppermint leaves, ⅓ cup of water, and 1 tablespoon of white cosmetic clay. Add the peppermint leaves and water to a blender and mix until green and frothy. Strain. In a small bowl, add mint liquid to the clay and stir until a spreadable paste forms. Spread onto a clean face and throat and let dry. Rinse.

Day 2: Zucchini Zit Zapper. This mask is alkaline, soothing, and chock-full of skin-healing minerals. It is good for inflamed, sensitive, oily, or acne-prone skin. Blend 1 baby zucchini, 3 or 4 inches long, with ¼ cup of water in your blender until smooth and pale green. Strain. In a coffee grinder or dry blender, grind 5 tablespoons of oatmeal until coarsely powdered (see the box on page 16). Save some of this powder for day 4. In a small bowl, mix sufficient zucchini liquid with 1 to 2 tablespoons of powdered oatmeal and let thicken for 1 minute. Spread this paste on your face and throat and allow to dry for 20 to 30 minutes. Rinse.

Day 3: Raspberry Fruit Acid Slougher. You may be tempted to drink this recipe rather than put it on your face! The natural fruit acids gently remove the outer layer of dead skin cells. The mixture may sting raw, sensitive, or sunburned skin; rinse off immediately if this occurs. Puree ⅓ cup of fresh, ripe raspberries in your blender or small food processor with a tablespoon of heavy cream, or mash together using a mortar and pestle. Apply this liquid with cotton ball to already-cleansed skin and leave on for 5 to 10 minutes. Rinse, then pat dry.

Day 4: Apple Juice and Red Wine Purification Pack. This recipe acts as a natural fruit acid skin slougher and pore refiner and helps to gradually even out your skin tone. Juice 1 fresh, small apple. If no fresh juice is available, chop the apple and put it in a blender with ¼ cup of water and puree; strain. In a small bowl, mix 2 teaspoons of fresh apple juice with 2 teaspoons of red wine and 1 scant tablespoon of ground oatmeal (see day 2) to make a spreadable paste. Add more liquid if necessary. Smooth onto a clean face and throat and let dry for 20 to 30 minutes. Rinse.

Day 5: Sage or Chamomile Softening Hair and Body Rinse. A multipurpose product! You'll need ½ cup of tightly packed and chopped fresh sage or whole chamomile flowers (sage for brunettes, chamomile for blondes and redheads), and 1 teaspoon of borax. Add these ingredients to a medium-size saucepan and pour in 6 cups of boiling water. Cover and steep for 15 minutes. Now add ½ cup of apple cider vinegar. Strain and cool. Use 1 cup as a final rinse after shampooing to soften and add sheen to your hair. Refrigerate leftovers for up to 10 days.

Hand Therapy

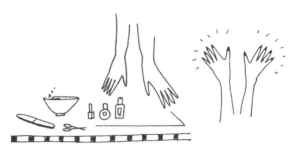

We tend to pay so much attention to our faces and hair but neglect one of our most expressive features, our hands. They are constantly exposed to the elements — sun, wind, heat, cold, harsh cleansers, dirt, grease — and are one of the first places on our bodies to show age.

Basic Hand Care

Apply moisturizer frequently throughout the day, especially after contact with water.

Wear rubber or latex gloves when exposed to water or cleansers, and wear quality cotton gardening gloves when working outdoors. Waterproof, cloth-lined gardening gloves are recommended when working with moist or soggy soil.

Get in the habit of applying a moisturizing sunscreen with a sun protection factor (SPF) of at least 15. Sun damage can result in premature aging of the skin, blotchiness, dryness, and the development of those dreaded "liver spots."

Banish onion, garlic, and tobacco odors from your hands by rubbing them with diluted lemon juice or apple cider vinegar. Or place a couple of drops of essential oil of orange on your palms and rub your hands together vigorously. Rinse with cool water and follow with an application of moisturizer.

To exfoliate dry skin from your hands, try this simple formula: In a small bowl, combine 1 tablespoon of sugar with 1 tablespoon of olive oil. Stir well. Now massage your hands thoroughly, especially around the cuticles and in between your fingers in the webbing. Rinse thoroughly and apply moisturizer.

To hydrate parched hands, apply to them a layer of moisturizing facial mask. Follow label directions for application and removal.

39

Improve Your Rear View

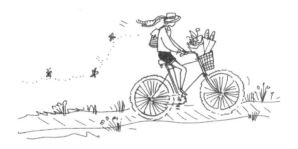

I f you're one of the few people who isn't afflicted with the lumps and bumps of cellulite, you're either very young or you've inherited one terrific set of genes. However, if you do have cellulite, there are several lifestyle "adjustments" you can make that will not only keep you healthier in general but also help prevent the formation or further development of cellulite.

Cellulite Treatment Tips

Get up, move, and sweat! Daily, vigorous aerobic exercise is paramount, so fight your sedentary tendencies. Try jogging, walking, dancing, bicycling, or in-line skating to stimulate circulation throughout your body, especially from the waist down (the area most commonly affected by cellulite).

Begin a regular aerobic weight-lifting routine to keep your underlying muscles toned and tight. It makes me really sweat and seems to carve the fat right off my thighs and buttocks as fast as a hot knife through butter. When I'm consistent about getting this type of exercise, I usually see results in as little as 10 days. Unfortunately, very few work-out tapes offer this type of exercise combination. Call your local gym to see if it offers classes.

Drink plenty of water. An ample intake of water will keep the toxins flowing right out of your body.

Eat a proper, balanced diet with as many whole, unrefined foods as possible. Reduce your consumption of refined and simple carbohydrates, including white flour, sugar and sugar substitutes, chips, cake, cookies, crackers, popcorn, and french fries, to name a few. Such starchy, sugary foods can cause weight gain and water retention.

Avoid salty foods like the plague! Salt causes your body to retain water, which can result in skin that looks puffy and bloated. This exacerbates the appearance of cellulite.

By all means stop smoking and avoid smoke-filled rooms. Smoking impairs circulation and adds poisonous toxins to your bloodstream.

Try yoga. If you've never taken a yoga-for-strength class, you may think that yoga is for people who can't do strenuous exercise. That assumption couldn't be farther from the truth. Yoga consists of performing a series of postures that strengthen your muscles and joints using your own body weight for resistance. I find that yoga tones and elongates my muscles, making for a leaner, more lithe look. It builds balance, coordination, and strength, and it's wonderfully de-stressing as well.

Dry-brush your skin every day. This is a wonderful technique for improving skin tone, circulation, and lymph flow, and for shedding dry skin. See Give Your Body the Brush-Off on page 109 for how-to instructions.

Keep alcohol and caffeine consumption to a minimum. They contribute more toxins for your body to deal with, and they sap your body of the nutrients essential for skin health.

Stay within your healthy weight range. Cellulite is more pronounced if you are overweight.

40

Eat for a Healthy Glow

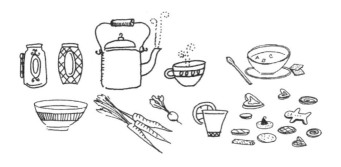

For a dreamy, creamy, clear complexion, proper nutrition is essential. Our skin needs many different nutrients to maintain a healthy pH balance and glowing appearance. The two recipes that follow are chock-full of easily absorbable vitamins and minerals. They'll also provide you with a delicious way to boost your energy levels as well as your natural immunity.

Skin-Sational Herb Tea

A tasty blend for an infusion that, hot or cold, helps replenish a deficient system and restore lackluster skin. All the herbs in this formula are in dried form. You'll get 25 to 30 cups of tea from this recipe.

> 2 tablespoons lemon balm leaves
> 1 tablespoon lavender flowers
> 1 tablespoon peppermint leaves
> 1 tablespoon chamomile flowers
> 1 tablespoon rose petals
> 1 tablespoon nettles
> 1 tablespoon alfalfa
> 1 tablespoon rose hips
> 2 teaspoons dandelion leaves
> 2 teaspoons raspberry leaves
> ½ teaspoon gingerroot

1. Combine all herbs in a medium-size bowl and stir to blend. Store in a tightly sealed tin, jar, or plastic tub or bag in a cool, dark location. Best if used within six months.

2. To use, bring a cup of water to a boil in a small saucepan. Remove from the heat and add 1 teaspoon of tea. Cover and allow to steep for 10 to 15 minutes.

3. Strain before drinking. Add honey or lemon if desired. You can consume up to three mugs daily.

Earth laughs in flowers.
— Ralph Waldo Emerson

Skin So Smoothie

I refer to this recipe as my "antistress breakfast boost" formula. It's loaded with complexion-enhancing, stress-reducing B vitamins, calcium, potassium, zinc, iron, fiber, protein, and complex carbohydrates for sustained energy. I love the taste, but if you're not crazy about brewer's yeast, the flavor will take a bit of getting used to. This formula makes enough for approximately two 1½-cup servings or one large meal.

  1 frozen banana or 1 cup frozen strawberries
  2 cups organic low-fat cow's milk or fortified soy milk
  1 tablespoon brewer's yeast
  2 teaspoons blackstrap molasses
  2 teaspoons raw sunflower seeds
  1 teaspoon raw sesame seeds
 10 raw almonds
  ¼ cup raw or cooked oatmeal
  2 teaspoons honey
  ¼ teaspoon ground cinnamon
 2–3 ice cubes (optional; makes a nice thick, frosty drink)

Combine all ingredients in a blender and mix on high until smooth, 30 to 60 seconds total. I usually consume the entire batch throughout the morning hours, taking sips between my work projects. You can also pour half of the mixture into a mug, cover, and refrigerate until later in the day.

Give Your Body the Brush-Off

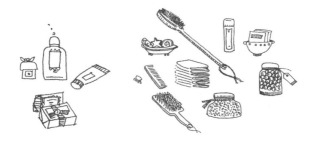

D ry, flaky skin is not only unsightly but uncomfortable, too. To eradicate dry skin, I recommend that both men and women adopt a simple yet invigorating morning ritual: dry-brushing, for epidermal stimulation. Dry-brushing revs up the circulation better than your morning cup-o-Joe, guaranteed. Perfect for those of you who suffer from winter "snake" skin.

Get Smooth and Healthy

Dry-brushing is a must for smooth, sleek, clear skin. Over the course of a day, your skin eliminates more than a pound of waste through thousands of tiny sweat glands. In fact, about one-third of all the body's impurities are excreted in this way.

If your pores are clogged by tight-fitting clothes, aluminum-containing antiperspirants, and mineral-oil-based moisturizers, there's no way for these toxic by-products to escape. Over time, the wastes build up, causing your skin to look pale, pasty, and pimply. The dead skin cells also build up on the epidermis, resulting in a dry, flaky, lizardlike texture that serves as a barrier impenetrable to most moisturizers. Ever keep applying moisturizer over and over again to your legs and arms yet still have that parched feeling, even though the bottle promises to alleviate even the most severely rough, dry skin? You have to get rid of the dead-cell buildup before the moisturizer can do any good! This is where dry-brushing lends a helping hand.

Contrary to what you might imagine, you can dry-brush over eczema and psoriasis. Granted, you may have to lighten up on your pressure a bit, but the stimulation is superb for those thickened, scaly, rough patches.

Repeat this ritual daily. It's a good idea to wash your body brush with soap and water every week or so to keep it free of skin debris.

Step 1: Dry-brushing is performed on dry skin — not oiled, not damp, but dry, before-you-bathe-or-shower skin. Using a natural-fiber brush the size of your palm, preferably one with a handle or strap, brush your entire body, except your face (and breasts, if you're a woman), for 5 to 10 minutes. Do not brush hard. Initially, you will have to start very

gently and work your way up to more vigorous brushing, but never scrub until you're red. Begin brushing your hands first, between the fingers, then the arms, underarms, neck, chest, stomach, sides, and back. Then brush each leg, beginning with the feet. You will feel wonderfully invigorated when you're finished, and your skin will glow!

Step 2: Now pour a tablespoon or so of sesame, almond, olive, or avocado oil into a small bowl and add a drop or two of lemongrass, basil, German chamomile, or lavender essential oil. Massage your entire body, including your face, ears, and scalp if you're washing your hair that day. Do this for about 5 minutes. Next, jump in the shower and bathe as normal; all of the dead skin you just exfoliated will be washed away. Be sure to pat, not rub, your skin dry, and apply a light moisturizer after you shower if necessary.

A DRY-BRUSH BONUS

Here's an added plus to dry-brushing: Because the process opens your clogged pores and aids in elimination, your cellulite will begin to diminish. Trust me; it works. Follow a good, low-fat diet and exercise program, and it will work even faster.

42

Nourish Your Nails

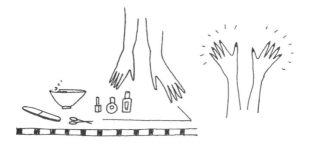

Nail problems that persist despite your consistent care can be a signal that something is lacking in your body. While some changes in appearance can be due to aging and climate, you should monitor your nails for signs of deeper problems. Your fingernails can suffer from brittleness, peeling, hangnails, weakness, ridges, discoloration, and spots if not fed the right foods. See your doctor if problems continue.

Fingernail Food

Nails are primarily composed of protein called keratin. Good sources of this essential nutrient include soy products, lean cuts of beef, poultry, fish, nuts, seeds, whole grains, beans, eggs, and yogurt.

If you're dieting, rapid weight loss can lead to nutritional deficiencies resulting in not-so-healthy, lackluster fingernails. Try to lose no more than 2 pounds per week and adhere to a balanced diet.

Stress zaps your body of iron and vitamins A, B, and C — necessary nutrients for strong, straight nails. It also reduces blood flow to your fingertips, leaving your nails looking pale.

Include in your diet foods such as pumpkin seeds and flaxseeds, and evening primrose or borage oils. These are rich in essential fatty acids that strengthen nails and moisturize surrounding skin.

Zinc, sulfur, and silica are important minerals known to fortify nails. Include broccoli, onions, garlic, spirulina, barley grass, alfalfa, dandelion, nuts, whole grains, and apples in your daily diet.

Biotin and folic acid, especially important B vitamins, help prevent and heal peeling, brittle nails.

A daily glass of calcium-rich carrot juice is a delicious way to strengthen bones, teeth, and nails. Calcium-fortified soy milk and skim cow's milk are also good sources.

43

Reflexology for Stress Relief

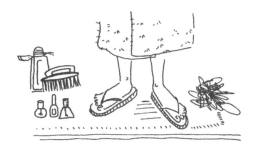

R eflexology is a science based on the idea that there are reflexes in the feet and hands relative to all the organs, functions, and parts of the human body. Applying pressure with your thumbs and forefingers to these points can bring about amazing results. Reflexology promotes stress relief, normalizes bodily functions, improves circulation, and relieves pain.

Let's Unwind

Your feet are actually more sensitive and receptive to touch than your hands because they contain a wealth of nerve endings, approximately 7,200 in each foot. Also, because they, unlike your hands, are not constantly exposed to the elements, they are highly responsive to the calming, tranquilizing effects induced by a reflexology session.

I can't possibly show you how to perform all of the various reflexology steps here. But the following are two basic reflexology techniques that can easily be performed at home to bring relief after a stressful day. Reflexology should always be practiced on a dry foot.

Big-Toe Stimulation: This exercise increases blood flow to your brain, pituitary and pineal glands, and neck. It also relieves neck stress and relaxes the mind. Holding the ball of your foot between your thumb (on the sole) and index fingers (on the top), "walk" down and "walk" up each of the five zones in your big toe. To find the zones, draw four evenly spaced vertical lines from the tip to the base of the big toe. In order to "thumb walk," you must make an inchwormlike motion with the outside edge of your thumb by bending the thumb repeatedly as you climb up or down, simultaneously applying pressure.

Solar Plexus Press: "The solar plexus is referred to as the 'nerve switchboard' of the body, as it is the main storage area for stress. Applying pressure to this reflex will always bring about a feeling of relaxation," say Inge Dougans and Suzanne Ellis, authors of *The Art of Reflexology.* To find the solar plexus reflex, grasp the top of your foot and gently squeeze the metatarsals (the five bones along the midportion of your foot that connect to each toe). A depression will have formed just under the ball of your foot and in the center. This depression represents the solar plexus reflex. Press your thumb into this spot and hold for a few seconds. Release. You can also work your thumb in small circular motions, first clockwise, then counterclockwise. Finish by pressing and holding again.

HEAL YOUR SKIN THROUGH STRESS REDUCTION

Skin disorders such as eczema, psoriasis, acne, hives, excess perspiration, and a pale complexion can be triggered or worsened by stress. Techniques for reducing stress include exercise, ample sleep, facial and body massage, reflexology, deep breathing, biofeedback, reiki, time with close friends and family, and recreation.

Make Your Bedroom a Haven

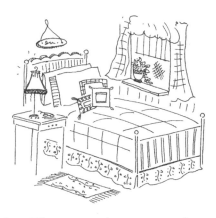

I t's a fact: The average human spends more time in the bedroom than any other room in the house, and frequently this room is designated for sleeping and nothing else. It doesn't have to be that way. Your bedroom should be your personal haven, with an ambience that is conducive to relaxation, meditation, reading, and romance.

Create a Private Retreat

F orget white walls — how boring! Experiment with color. If you're timid, try a pastel shade first; if you're more dramatic, try a bolder color. Use your imagination!

Plants can add serenity and interest to a bedroom, not to mention oxygenating the air and adding a natural look. If your furnishings are sparse, plant a large palm, benjamin ficus, or rubber tree in a decorative pot and place it in front of a big sunny window. Take care to keep it out of reach of children and pets.

If your bedroom is spacious enough to accommodate a chair and ottoman or a chaise lounge, then by all means invest in one. These chairs offer the utmost in comfort and actually provide a come-hither invitation to recline and read or nap.

Invest in high-quality flannel, pima cotton, or satin sheets. Sleeping should be as cozy or sensual as possible.

Keep a daily journal on your nightstand. Each night, pause and write down your reflections of the day. It's a good way to unwind and allow the day's business to drain away.

Keep a tea tray next to your bed or chair and stock it with your favorite herbal or regular teas. Fill a beautiful ceramic or pottery teapot with boiling water, bring it into your bedroom, and brew a pot of relaxation.

Place several scented candles of varying heights in front of a mirror, perhaps on your dresser. Light them before a romantic encounter to scent the air, and watch the light flicker and dance.

Rediscover the joys of an imaginative journey through reading. Keep a selection of soul-nourishing books at your bedside.

Make or purchase several velvet or chenille throw pillows that coordinate with your bedroom colors. They're cushy and soft and make a great back support for reading in bed.

Designate a special area in your bedroom for practicing yoga, meditation, or simple stretching exercises. These are wonderful ways to ease into or end your day.

Finally, don't forget music. It can calm you down, rev you up, make you feel like dancing or singing, wake you up, or lull you to sleep.

45

Surround Yourself with Fragrance

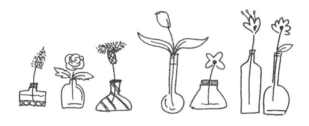

Because fragrance so strongly touches the brain's emotional centers, it can dramatically affect mood and memory. Fresh-baked chocolate chip cookies, an evergreen forest in summer, an ocean breeze, a newborn puppy — all evoke wonderful memories that can be rekindled in an instant at the first whiff of the scent.

Stop and Smell the Roses

My favorite fragrant flowers are the double rosa rugosa, lilac, lavender, honeysuckle, wild azalea, hyacinth, privet, gardenia, lily-of-the-valley, freesia, rose, verbena, and orange blossom. This mixture of shrubs, bushes, perennials, and vines produces flowers with intense, heady, intoxicatingly sweet aromas.

To scent your percale sheets and make them feel more like silk, sprinkle with a light dusting of your favorite perfumed dusting powder.

Need an instant, cooling energy boost? Spray the soles of your feet with chilled cologne or chilled peppermint or rose geranium herbal water.

Place a cake of your favorite perfumed soap into your lingerie drawer — or your desk at work, for that matter. Every time you open the drawer, you'll receive a waft of fragrance.

Citrusy Room Freshener

Essential oils of grapefruit and lemon combine to make a light, sweet, refreshing spray that will simultaneously neutralize any unpleasant smells (especially pet odors) while lifting your spirits. Economical and chemical-free!

   ½ cup distilled water
   1 teaspoon essential oil of lemon
   1 teaspoon essential oil of grapefruit

Pour the blend into a 4-ounce glass mister. Shake well before using to mist the air throughout your home.

46

Mask Yourself

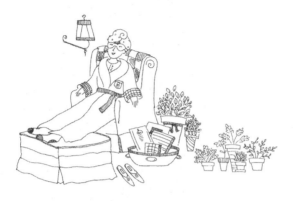

Facial masks can be made from myriad natural ingredients and are used to deep-clean, tone, exfoliate, or soften the skin, or to stimulate a sluggish complexion. Masks should always be applied to freshly cleansed, damp skin. Try to lie or sit down and rest while using the mask; relaxation will only further the benefits of the treatment.

Uncover the Real You

To reestablish that "peaches and cream" glow in normal, dry, or highly sensitive skin, mash half of a very ripe, small peach with 2 teaspoons of heavy cream. Apply the paste to your face and neck and leave on for 30 minutes. Rinse with warm water.

Need an instant mask that's calming and soothing for sunburned or irritated skin that's either normal or oily? Grab the bottle of milk of magnesia from the medicine chest and apply it in a thin layer over your entire face, throat, and chest. Let it dry for 5 to 10 minutes. Rinse with warm water. Follow with a light moisturizer.

An apple a day keeps dry-skin buildup away! Apples contain malic acid, a mild alpha-hydroxy acid that sloughs off the surface layer of dead skin cells. In the blender, mix half of a small peeled apple with a tiny amount of water until smooth. Apply the pulpy liquid with a cotton ball to your face, throat, and chest. Allow to dry for 15 to 20 minutes. Rinse with warm water. This mask can be used by all skin types.

Brewer's Yeast Circulation Booster

This mask can be used by all skin types. It brings a very rosy glow to the skin and helps chase away that winter "pasty" look.

- 1 tablespoon brewer's yeast
- 2 teaspoons water (oily skin), 1 or 2 percent milk (normal skin), or cream (dry skin)

Combine the ingredients to form a smooth paste. You may need more or less liquid than called for, depending on the brand of yeast. Spread this onto your face and throat in a thin layer; let dry. Rinse. This mask may tingle as it dries, which is normal. If it starts to sting, rinse it off immediately and follow with a good moisturizer.

47

Tips for Luscious Lips

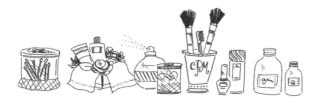

Your lips, unlike the rest of your skin, contain no sebaceous (oil) glands or sweat glands and therefore cannot moisturize themselves. If lip tissue is damaged by heat, cold, drying lipsticks, smoking, too many happy-hour beverages, herpes, or other agents, the small amount of saliva that reaches your lips via the tip of the tongue will not be sufficient to prevent your lips from becoming dehydrated.

Pucker Up!

When venturing out into the sun, be it the beach or bright ski slope, don't forget to apply a lip balm with an SPF of 15 or higher.

Thick castor oil, an ingredient in lipstick, can be applied straight out of the bottle for a glossy look.

Slick on a bit of cocoa butter for a moisturizing, chocolate-flavored lip treat. Great for men and boys because it's colorless and not too shiny.

After brushing your teeth, gently brush your lips as well. "Not only does it take away any chapping, but it plumps up the lip temporarily for that sought-after 'pouty' look," says Diane Irons, author of *The World's Best-Kept Beauty Secrets.*

Apply a lip balm frequently throughout the day to create a moisture-resistant barrier on your lips that will help prevent moisture loss.

Keep hydrated! Make sure to drink lots of water throughout the day.

A dab of honey on your lips will act as a humectant, drawing moisture from the air to your skin, keeping your lips soft, plump, and kissably sweet.

A dab of vegetable glycerin mixed with vitamin E or wheat germ oil makes an effective, nourishing moisture barrier.

48

Learn to Love Lavender

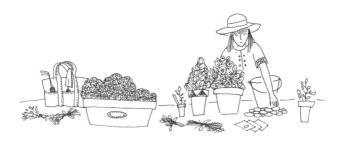

From ancient Greece to modern times, lavender has been one of the most common and widely used cultivated herbs. And it's no wonder, because it's one of the most versatile, too. All forms of lavender — essential oil, dried or fresh flowers, aromatic hydrosol, and tea — are safe to use on all skin types, even young children's delicate skin.

The Benefits of Lavender

Grow a patch of lavender. Plant a few mounds in a sunny spot around a garden bench or large stone or log. On a hot summer's day, have a seat in your lavender patch. Brush your hands against the plant and inhale the delightful scent wafting through the breeze. Lavender is recommended for people who experience constant stress and overstimulation and find it difficult to relax and unwind.

The essential oil of these lovely, purple, highly fragrant flowers can soothe your soul without sapping your energy. To enhance concentration and promote mental clarity, place a drop on your wrist, the palms of your hands, or the nape of your neck and breathe deeply.

Lavender is a potent antiseptic. Add 2 drops of essential oil of lavender to 1 teaspoon of soybean, almond, olive, or hazelnut oil or aloe vera juice and apply the mixture directly to burns, sunburns, abrasions, insect stings, or inflamed pimples to cleanse and disinfect.

Make a skin-softening bath sachet. Combine ¼ cup dried lavender flowers, ¼ cup instant, powdered whole milk, and ¼ cup oatmeal. Place into a 3-by-5-inch muslin drawstring bag. Toss the bag into the bathwater so that the ingredients can release their skin-pampering properties. Rub the sachet over your entire body to cleanse and hydrate dry skin.

Improve your mood. Purchase a bottle of lavender aromatic hydrosol — a watery by-product of essential oil distillation — and spray a fine mist onto your face and hair, and into the surrounding air. Inhale the vapors. The chemical components of the lavender plant have the ability to alter the emotions by influencing the sense of smell, which triggers the region of the brain that deals with memory and mood.

Old-Fashioned Lavender Vinegar

Sprinkle a dash of this fragrant vinegar onto a salad for a delectable departure from your ordinary dressing, or use 1 part vinegar to 8 parts water as a facial toner or hair rinse. This recipe makes approximately 2 cups of vinegar.

- 1 cup fresh or ½ cup dried lavender flowers and leaves
- 2 teaspoons lemon zest
- 2 cups raw apple cider vinegar

Place the lavender and lemon zest in a clean quart-size canning jar and pour in the unheated vinegar. Cover the top with plastic wrap, then screw on the lid and store in a dark, cool place for two to four weeks. Shake daily. Strain the vinegar, bottle in a decorative container, and use as you would ordinary vinegar.

Happy is he who hath the power to gather wisdom from a flower.

— **Anonymous**

49

Make an Herbal Dream Pillow

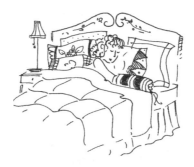

A dream pillow is a fragrant, soft little pillow filled with the herbs traditionally used to calm nightmares; evoke colorful, exotic, or peaceful dreams; or simply help you sleep more soundly. Tuck a pillow into your pillowcase while you sleep and let the fairies and dream weavers lead you into the land of Nod.

Choose your favorite mixture and follow the instructions below for making a dream pillow. All herbs used are in dried form, unless stated otherwise.

Scented Slumber

For Soothing, Outdoor Dreams: ¼ cup fresh or dried spruce or balsam fir needles, ¼ cup fresh or dried pine needles cut into ½-inch pieces, ¼ cup mugwort, ¼ cup lemon balm.

For Romantic Dreams: ¼ cup lavender, ¼ cup rose petals, ¼ cup whole chamomile, 2 table-spoons hops, and 2 tablespoons catnip. If you have cats, you might want to omit the catnip; my cat, Toby, discovered this particular flannel-encased pillow and took it away for his own bed!

For Vivid, Colorful Dreams: ½ cup lemongrass, ¼ cup marigold flowers, ¼ cup mugwort.

Dream Pillow

This pillow is easy to make and perfect for gift giving. Sweet dreams!

Choose one of the above blends or create your own favorite mixture

1. To make a quick pillow, buy a 3-by-5-inch or 4-by-6-inch plain, muslin cloth drawstring bag and fill it with your herbs. Tie closed. You can also use the plain bag as the liner and cover it in a softer, more decorative fabric such as flannel, silk, satin, or velveteen.

2. To make your own custom pillow cover, cut an 11-inch square piece of fabric and hem the raw edges to ½ inch with stitching.

3. Place the herb-filled liner bag onto the wrong side of the decorative fabric and wrap the bag like a piece of hard candy. Tie both ends of the fabric with a piece of ribbon. Refill the herb liner every two or three months.

50

Words of Wisdom

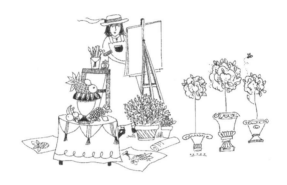

There are a multitude of self-help books out there to treat the mind, body, and spirit. But sometimes the most important concepts to remember are the simplest: lessons you learned from your parents, teachers, children, or even your own experiences. Take the time to appreciate what you have and recall a few wise words that will inspire you throughout the day.

Live Well

Trust in yourself. Your creativity will flow and life will be easier to handle.

Raise your energy level and ability to concentrate by practicing deep breathing. Breathe in deeply and exhale completely.

Exercise on a regular basis.

Bathe weekly in your favorite essential oils.

Eat more fresh fruits and vegetables.

Choose challenge and change.

Ask for hugs from those you love.

Do something that will make you feel good about yourself; have a massage, buy yourself a special treat, or take a day off.

Talk to and love the child inside you.

Stop blaming yourself and others.

Begin each day on a positive note. Buy a book of

daily devotions or inspirational mottos and read
one every morning when you arise.

Ask someone you trust to tell you what they like
about you.

Communicate with nature. Take walks, explore
the nearby woods, or even just sit outside on the
grass and appreciate the sights, sounds, and smells.

Sit quietly and listen to your heart; it often gives
the best advice.

SELF-AFFIRMATIONS

Practice self-affirmations every day to keep
your perspective positive and uplifting. Here
are some examples:

* "I now trust myself completely."

* "I am a smart and talented go-getter."

* "I am calm and relaxed no matter what the
  circumstances."

* "I am at peace."

* "I will not worry, no matter what comes
  my way today."

* "I can do anything I set my mind to."

Index

Other Storey Titles You Will Enjoy

The Essential Oils Book, by Colleen K. Dodt. A rich resource on the many applications of aromatherapy and its uses in everyday life. 160 pages. Paperback. ISBN 0-88266-913-3.

The Herbal Body Book, by Stephanie Tourles. Learn how to transform common herbs, fruits, and grains into safe, economical, and natural personal care items. Contains over 100 recipes to make facial scrubs, hair rinses, shampoos, soaps, cleansing lotions, moisturizers, lip balms, toothpaste, powders, insect repellents, and more. 128 pages. Paperback. ISBN 0-88266-880-3.

The Herbal Home Spa, by Greta Breedlove. These easy-to-make recipes include facial steams, scrubs, masks, and lip balms; massage oils, baths, rubs, and wraps; hand, nail, and foot treatments; and shampoos, dyes, and conditioners. Relaxing bathing rituals and massage techniques are also covered. 208 pages. Paperback. ISBN 0-88266-005-6.

Natural Foot Care, by Stephanie Tourles. From easy-to-make recipes for creams, lotions, and ointments, to foot massage techniques, this book offers dozens of natural ways to care for feet. 192 pages. Paperback. ISBN 1-58017-054-4.

Natural Hand Care, by Norma Pasekoff Weinberg. Focusing on alternative and preventive therapies and treatments, this book offers dozens of easy-to-make recipes for cosmetic products, plus nutrition tips for healthy hands, strength-building exercises, and relaxing hand-massage techniques. 272 pages. Paperback. ISBN 1-58017-053-6.

Rosemary Gladstar's Herbs for Natural Beauty, by Rosemary Gladstar. This self-affirming book includes Gladstar's own 5-Step Program for Perfect Skin, and includes her personal formulations for herbal steams, cleansers, astringents, and creams. She also explores the therapeutic and beauty benefits of herbal baths, bath salts, and massage oils, and offers recipes for shampoos, conditioners, and henna tints. 80 pages. Paperback. ISBN 1-58017-152-4.